A COMPEND OF THE PRINCIPLES OF HOMEOPATHY

As Taught By Hahnemann And Verified By A Century Of Clinical Application

William Boericke

GYAN

Published by

Gyan Publishing House
5, Ansari Road
Daryaganj, New Delhi-110002
Phone: 011-47034999, 9811692060
E-mail: books@gyanbooks.com

Distribution Network
gyanbooks.com
India, USA, Canada, UK, Australia

ISBN: 978-93-6208-179-7 (HB)
First Published, 1896

2nd Impression 2024

Printed at: Gyan Press, Delhi.

A COMPEND OF THE PRINCIPLES OF HOMEOPATHY
Author: WILLIAM BOERICKE

A COMPEND

OF THE

Principles of Homœopathy

AS TAUGHT BY HAHNEMANN,
AND VERIFIED BY A CENTURY OF CLINICAL APPLICATION,

— BY —

WM. BOERICKE, M. D.

Professor of Materia Medica and Therapeutics, at the Hahnemann Hospital College of San Francisco; Associate Author of the Twelve Tissue Remedies of Schuessler; Stepping Stone to Homœopathy; Member of American Institute of Homœopathy, Etc., Etc.

SAN FRANCISCO:
BOERICKE & RUNYON,
1896.

PREFACE.

Hahnemann's Organon is the great text-book of the homœopathic school. It contains philosophical conceptions and practical directions for the establishment of a true science of therapeutics, and all genuine progress towards this goal is in the direction pointed out in that work. To fix its principles clearly in the mind of the student, to faithfully apply them in practice, is the special duty and high privilege of Homœopathy. The more this is done, the more will this masterly book become a veritable mountain of therapeutic light to the practitioner.

Hahnemann's teachings, and the therapeutic edifice erected by the homœopathic school, are based upon two distinct factors. On the one hand, upon facts of observation and experiment obtained by strict adherence to the inductive methods of research, facts that can thus be verified at all times; and, on the other hand, upon new ideas resulting from the exercise of deductive reasoning, ideas belonging possibly to a larger and higher realm, and to some extent beyond the acceptance of modern scientific thought, but nevertheless capable of great power in achieving curative results.

Until quite recently, the tendency of modern homœopathy was to bend its energies perhaps too exclusively upon the acquisition of the facts yielding immediate results, while neglecting to some extent the study of the underlying principles. With neglect of the study of homœopathic institutes came coquetry with old-school methods, and the alluring adoption of modern palliative and mechanical therapeutics, leading unquestionably to deterioration of our distinctive practice. The reaction had to come. We are in the midst of it. A homœopathic renaissance is upon us. Teach and study the Organon is its watchword. This little book is intended to be an introduction and an aid to a fuller study and wider acceptance of Hahnemann's doctrines. It does not pretend to be more than an attempt to elucidate the salient and vital points often abstrusely and always metaphorically treated by Hahnemann, and thus to familiarize the student with the fundamental groundwork of our school. These essential doctrines do not include the necessary acceptance of every statement of Hahnemann as of equal and absolute importance. Indeed, a wise discrimination is necessary, for the minor things may be instructive or obstructive, or even destructive, according to the way they are held; they may, therefore, be useful or otherwise for the mental development of the physician or the scientific evolution of the school.

The author has gladly availed himself of everything published that furthered the end in view, and he hopes that the little volume will be used by the student and young practitioner as a first stepping-stone to the rich mine of deep philosophy and practical suggestion contained in the writings of Samuel Hahnemann.

WM. BOERICKE, M. D.

SAN FRANCISCO, SEPTEMBER, 1896.

CONTENTS.

CHAPTER IV.

DRUG-PROVING.

CHAPTER V.

INTERPRETATION OF DRUG PATHOGENESIS.

CHAPTER VI.

DRUG RELATIONSHIP.

CHAPTER VII.

THE APPLICATION OF HOMŒOPATHY.

CHAPTER VIII.

THE SIMILIMUM.

CHAPTER IX.

THE SECOND PRESCRIPTION.

CHAPTER X.

HAHNEMANN'S NOSOLOGY.

CHAPTER XI.

CHAPTER XII.

CHAPTER XIII.

APPENDIX.

A COMPEND

OF THE

PRINCIPLES OF HOMŒOPATHY.

CHAPTER I.

THE THERAPEUTIC FIELD.

The aim of the art of medicine is to cure disease, and the physician's highest ideal of a cure, as Hahnemann says, Organon § 2, is the rapid, gentle and permanent restoration of health, or the removal and annihilation of disease in its whole extent, in the shortest, most reliable and most harmless manner, and on easily comprehensible principles, that is, with the least possible expenditure of time, money, vitality and suffering.

In pursuance of this object, the physician presses into his service all agencies which tend to health. This is the part of

Therapeutics [*therapeuein*, to attend upon]. It includes all that relates to the science and art of healing, includes all agents, medicines among them, which may aid this purpose. It embraces dietetics, climate, clothing, bathing, nursing, application of heat, cold, electricity and all other means used by the physician for restoring health, when that is possible, or in palliating violent conditions or incurable diseases, or in preventing their development. Hence there are

Three methods of combating disease, of which every physician is bound to avail himself. They are:

1. Preventive medicine.
2. Palliative medicine.
3. Curative medicine.

These cover the whole field of possible therapeutic activity.*

Preventive Medicine includes the application of everything that physiology, hygiene, sanitary science, etc., can teach to lessen the development of disease according to the teaching in § 4 of the Organon.

"The physician is at the same time a preserver of health, when he knows the causes that disturb health, that produce and maintain disease, and when he knows how to remove them from healthy persons."

It includes much of bacteriological knowledge, antiseptic medication, subjects that have made enormous strides in recent years. It includes as well the judicious use of homœopathic remedies in preventing or modifying the development of epidemic and hereditary diseases.

Palliative Medicine. Palliative medicines are of two kinds:

(1) The use of drugs in their physiological dosage for their direct effects, as the use of Opium and Morphine for pain. This is the common method of the old school.

(2) By the carefully selected Homœopathic remedy given in minute dosage. This frequently yields brilliant results in palliating where a cure is impossible. This latter method is to be tried in every case before *drug* palliation is used.

This is almost the sole resource of the old school, and consequently much abused, but in the hands of the

---

*This was aptly and perfectly expressed by Dr. Hering to the author in the German words *Hindern, Lindern, Mindern*, embodying every possibility of a physician's distinctive sphere of usefulness.

true physician who knows its subordinate place, it constitutes a legitimate method in incurable diseases, beyond the operation of the law of cure, where we can only alleviate, not radically cure. While Homœopathy reduces the need and occasions for the use of mere palliatives to a small limit, yet palliation has its use in the practice of medicine, but it is always the expression on the part of the physician of his impotence to cure radically.

Curative Medicine is almost exclusively occupied by Homœopathy, for this method alone cures without subjecting the patient to new pains and discomforts; it alone fulfills the highest aim of the physician—to heal quickly, gently, radically, according to scientific and rational methods.

All physicians are compelled to avail themselves of all three methods at times. As sanitarians and hygienists, physicians can do much to prevent zymotic and epidemic diseases; as homœopathists, much can be done in the eradication of inherited disease tendencies and preventing their development; and as the laws that govern curative medicine are applied more fully, the need for mere palliation will correspondingly grow less.

Leaving aside the large field of General Therapeutics, common to all physicians, of whatever school of medicine, we restrict ourselves to the consideration of the different uses of drugs as therapeutic agents.

Medicinal Therapeutics is the application of drugs as medicines for the purpose of modifying or curing disease. Drugs are employed in the medicinal therapeutic field either empirically, or according to the Law of Similars—i. e., scientifically, because according to fixed law.

Empiricism is based upon mere experience and is practice without regard to any theory or scientific deduction or investigation. A remedy is given which experience has shown to be effective in a similar case. It is the rule of authority and leads to mechanical routinism in practice. Certain remedies have, however, obtained a permanent place in medicine that have been discovered empirically, and whose mode of action cannot be readily explained. It has been found that certain drugs act curatively against certain definite diseases when given in material dosage. They are known as specifics. There are not many, but such are Quinine in malaria, Mercury in syphilis, Iodine in glandular affections, Salicylic acid in rheumatism, etc. These occupy a rather unique position, though it can be claimed that the relationship is a homœopathic one, although it differs from the usual homœopathic relationship between remedies to disease in requiring material dosage.

Practice according to some pathological theory is characteristic of the old school of medicine. It is constantly changing, as different views on physiology and pathology lead to corresponding therapeutic changes. It is therefore one of the most unstable of methods. At present, pathology being dominated by bacteriological views, the corresponding therapeutic measures are largely germicidal, anti-septic or anti-toxical. But already bacterial pathology, and as a consequence its therapeutics show signs of the inevitable displacement.*

The use of medicines when administered according to some pathological theory is either according to allopathic or antipathic method.

---

*Says Lawson Tait, that during his professional life he has learned and unlearned some four or five theories of inflammation, and he predicts that the present prevalent theory, coccophobia he calls it, will soon go the way of the other theories.

Allopathy (from *Allos*, other and *Pathos*, a disease), where the symptoms are different, the same organs and tissues being affected in a different manner, or other organs and tissues being affected in some manner; the relationship being one of *indefinite diversity**

Allopathy usually attacks the parts most exempt from the disease, in order to draw away the disease through them and thus to expel it, as is imagined. § 55 Organon.

Antipathy, or **Eantiopathy** (from *Eanthios*, contrary, and *Pathos*, disease)—where the symptoms, or conditions indicated by them, are opposites; the relationship being one of *direct antagonism*. It is a palliative method, pure and simple, wherewith the physician can *appear* to be most useful and can usually gain the patient's confidence by deluding him with momentary amelioration.

The inefficacy and danger of this method as applied in diseases of a chronic nature is easily verified by clinical observation. Study § 56–71 Organon.

"All pure experience and exact experiment will convince us that persistent symptoms of disease are so imperfectly alleviated or exterminated by *contrary* symptoms of a drug, used according to antipathic or palliative method, that after a brief period of apparent relief, they will break forth again in a more marked degree, and visibly aggravated." Organon § 23.

In this category of allopathic treatment belong the therapeutic method of Biochemistry, introduced by Dr. Schuessler of Germany, and the various forms of chemical treatment, such as Hensel's, etc. The former adopted from Homœopathy its method of diminishing dosage and some of its distinctive remedies, but other-

---

*Dake, Pathogenetic Therapeutics.

wise it has no relationship to Homœopathy, since its therapeutic procedures are based upon a *pathological theory* and not upon the symptoms of the individual patient, which alone constitute the basis of homœopathic therapeutics. Here also belongs

Organo-Therapy, which is that therapeutic method which aims to supply deficiencies in the functional activity of human organs by the administration of substances derived from similar organs in animals.

It has been found that the extract of Thyroid gland of animals, administered to the human organism, causes a rapid disappearance of the morbid symptoms of myxedema—a form of disease or atrophy of the thyroid, interfering with the performance of its function.

The doctrine that sound organs of certain animals are useful in diseases of those organs in man so lately revived in the old school, was clearly taught by Oswald Croll, a disciple of Paracelsus. Its modern extension is unreasonable and unscientific, and a passing therapeutic fad.

Besides these special and modern tendencies of old school practice, there are certain perennial features characteristic of it. In place of the former hypothetical assumptions of the hidden causes of disease that proved delusive and deceptive as a basis for treatment, material causes of disease were next assumed to exist, and hence the treatment, based upon such hypotheses, consisted mostly in eliminating from the organism the supposed offending cause, therefore the list of purgatives, emetics, sudorifics counter-irritants, surgical procedures, local medication of all kinds. But though a temporary relief is frequently obtained thereby, no permanent cure is established, rather an increase in the very condition, in the case of chronic disease; or metastases appear sooner or later, which, however, are then looked upon as new diseases, and not as direct results of ill-adapted treatment.

"But in by far the greatest proportion of cases of disease, known as chronic, these impetuous, weakening, and indirect therapeutie measures of the old school scarcely ever prove to be of the least benefit. For a few days at most they suspend one or another of those troublesome manifestations of disease which return, however, as soon as nature has become inured to that counter-stimulus; and the disease will re-appear with more violence, because the vital powers have been reduced by the pain of counter-irritation and improper evacuations." *

Objections to Antipathic Treatment.

(1) It is merely symptomatic treatment attacking some prominent single condition, instead of the disease as a whole, and necessarily leads to polypharmacy in the endeavor to meet different conditions at the same time.

(2) The transient amelioration is followed by an increased aggravation of the very condition to be removed, necessitating increasing dosage.

(3) Drug diseases are established that complicate hopelessly the original disease of the patient; the possibility of harm by the introduction of the necessary large dosage of drugs and foreign substances always being very evident.

None of these therapeutic methods are curative in the true sense by directly modifying the vital activities of the organism. In the cases where such treatment is ultimately successful (and certain temporary beneficial results cannot be denied), the homœopathic method is more direct, safer, more radical, and with no possible harm to the patient.

* "Organon," Introduction.

Practice based upon the Law of Cure is the only truly scientific therapeutic method, since it alone fulfills the conditions of science and offers a medical practice true for all time and applicable to all forms of disease in men and animals.

Homœopathy is the only therapeutic method based upon law.

Similia Similibus Curantur.* Like affections are cured by their similars, expresses the law for drug selection in all curable forms of disease. By its application, the curative remedy is found in curable cases; and in incurable cases, the same law usually points to a remedy that will act palliatively in most conditions. By Law of Cure is meant the definite path along which a drug force moves to cure a diseased condition. This law forms the basis of Homœopathy [from the Greek words *homoios* and *pathos*, meaning similar affections], the therapeutic method that applies the principle that any drug which is capable of pro-

---

* There exists a misconception concerning the phraseology employed by Hahnemann in the expression of the Law of Similars. Dr. R. E. Dudgeon, the recognized authority concerning the works of Hahnemann, writes in the appendix to his translation of the Organon, "Hahnemann always wrote the formula **Similia Similibus Curentur**, thereby giving an imperative or mandatory turn to the phrase." The translation must evidently be "Let likes be treated by likes." "*Durch Beobachtung, Nachdenken und Erfahrung fand ich, dass im Gegentheile von letzlern* [*Erleichterungsmittel und Palliative durch die Curart contraria contrariis*] *die wahre, richtige, beste Heilung zu finden sei in dem Satze* **Similia Similibus Curentur.** *Wähle, um sanft, schnell, gewiss und dauerhaft zu heilen, in jedem Krankheitsfalle eine Argnei, welche ein aehnliches Leiden für sich erregen kann, als sie heilen soll!*" Nevertheless, Similia Similibus **Curantur** has been almost universally adopted by the homœopathic school, and the belief and conviction have been unconsciously expressed thereby that it is a *law of nature*—S. S. Curantur—Likes are cured by likes; rather than a rule of art, S. S. Curentur—Let likes be treated by likes.

ducing symptoms of disease in the healthy will remove similar symptoms, and thus cure the disease when found in the sick.

The first promulgation of this principle was made by Hahnemann in 1796, in an essay published in Hufeland's Journal, entitled "On a new principle for ascertaining the curative properties of drugs." In this essay Hahnemann formulated his conclusions thus: "Every powerful medicinal substance produces in the human body a peculiar kind of disease, the more powerful the medicine, the more peculiar, marked and violent the disease. We should imitate nature, which sometimes cures a chronic disease by superadding another and employ in the disease we wish to cure *that* medicine which is able to produce another very similar artificial disease, and the former will be cured—Similia Similibus."

This was six years after his first experiments with Cinchona bark, which was the first drug experimented with and which gave striking evidences of the similarity between the effects it is capable of producing, and those for which it had ever been employed, and which was the beginning of a rational, scientific, Materia Medica, and of a scientific therapeutics based thereon. The most characteristic feature about the development of Homœopathy is the strict observance of the inductive method of research that Hahnemann adopted. Careful experiments were instituted, all preconceived theories were ostracized, and the results and rigid deduction from them were not published until years had elapsed in which to verify all the statements.

The development of the homœopathic principle began in the mind of Hahnemann with his experiments with Cinchona, which in turn led him to other experiments with other drugs and patient search of recorded action and uses of drugs throughout the medical literature. His first suggestions fell unheeded by the profession; but he continued his experiments, and nine years later published a work in Latin "On the Positive Effects of Medicines," and at the same time declared the principle of Similars as a law of general application. Five years more of further reflection and experiment enabled him to perfect his system and embody its principles in his great book, the "Organon of Rational Medicine." The following year, while a teacher at the University of Leipsic, he published volume I of his "Materia Medica Pura," containing original provings made by himself and members of his family, and assisted later by some enthusiastic disciples that gathered around him at the University; and in 1821 he published the final sixth volume, containing the positive effects of sixty-four medicines. With the publication of these two great works, Hahnemann provided both the theoretical and practical requirements of Homœopathy as a distinct method of therapeutics. He was the first to apply the inductive method of research to therapeutics. He says, in the preface to the second edition of the Organon, published in 1818: "The true healing art is in its nature a pure science of experience, and can and must rest on clear facts and on the sensible phenomena pertaining to their sphere of action. Its subjects can only be derived from pure experience and observation, and it dares not take a single step out of the sphere of pure, well-observed experience and experiment." And, again, "Every one of its conclusions about the actual must *always* be based on sensible perceptions, facts and experiences, if it would elicit the truth."

Homœopathy, the Science of Therapeutics. Such a healing art conformable to nature and experience, a science of therapeutics, therefore, did not exist before Hahnemann.

The most marked feature of the early homœopathy was its entire freedom from all theory and hypothesis; it was a protest against all and any pathological theory *as a basis of therapeutics.*

As taught, it was the true science of therapeutics, based upon exact observation of natural phenomena in disease and drug action, and noting the law governing their mutual relationship.

On this solid ground of scientific observation, all Homœopathists base their practice, whatever differences have arisen, date from the publication of Hahnemann's theory of chronic diseases and drug dynamization, and in not clearly distinguishing between Hahnemann's discoveries and facts on the one hand and his illustrations and mere theories on the other. Whatever Hahnemann published as a fact has never yet been disproved, but his theories are not proven. It is the genuine Hahnemannian spirit, as Hering says, totally to disregard all theories, even those of one's own fabrication, when they are in opposition to the results of pure experience. All theories and hypotheses have no positive weight whatever, only so far as they lead to new experiments and afford a better survey of the results of those already made.

The Great Central Truths of Homœopathy.

(1) The totality of symptoms of the patient constitutes the disease for the purpose of a cure.

(2) Drug experimentation on the healthy, so-called drug proving, is the only reliable method to arrive at a knowledge of the effects of drugs.

(3) The curative relation between these two sets of symptomatic facts is the law of similars, Similia Similibus Curantur.

(4) The administration of one single remedy at a time.

(5) The minimum (smallest) dose that will bring about a cure.

(6) Repetition of the dose should cease when marked improvement sets in.

Isopathic Medication and its modern form of Serum-Therapy. This means the employment of morbid products of a disease for the cure of the same disease [Aequalia aequalibus]. It is of very ancient date, and of late has received renewed attention through the researches of Pasteur, Koch, and others; it necessitates the attenuation of the virus, in order to be used medicinally; it was taught as early as 400 years B. C. by Xenocrates; it was introduced into Homœopathy by Dr. Lux in 1823, and in part adopted by Dr. Hering. Lux taught that the toxins formed in the body, properly attenuated, are capable of curing the very diseases that give rise to them—that is, every disease is supposed to have within itself its own antidoté.

In 1830 Hering proposed as a remedy for hydrophobia the saliva of a rabid dog, properly attenuated; the very teaching and practice of Pasteur. He also proposed Phthisine as a remedy for tuberculosis, and forty years later it, too, received popular and scientific endorsement by Koch and others. As early as 1834, Dr. Stapf, one of the greatest of the early homœopathists, who looked upon the subject dispassionately, says: "I do not doubt that the discovery of the curative action of morbid matters, in diseases that produced them, to be one of the most important discoveries that has been made since the beginning of our school."

Nosodes is the homœopathic designation for such morbid products, which are animal alkaloids [ptomaines], produced by the decomposition of animal substances. At first ptomaines were restricted to alkaloids produced by cadaveric decomposition, hence the name (ptomaine, belonging to a dead body), but now they also include alkaloids of animal origin formed during life as a result of chemical changes within the organism. These alkaloids have assumed great importance, by reason of their relation to the causation of disease, and it is probable that most pathogenic bacteria produce their effects *through their specific alkaloids.* The homœopathic nosodes are these specific alkaloids attenuated according to homœopathic methods and administered according to the Law of Similars. To obtain a permanent place in the Materia Medica, as Psorinum, the principal of the nosodes, has already achieved, and not be the victim of a passing therapeutic fad, as is the fate of most old-school therapeutic novelties, *they must be proved on the healthy,* and the pathogenetic effects thus obtained be the only guide for their therapeutic application. To apply them empirically for similar *diseases* corresponding to their origin as is done by the old-school with tuberculin, antitoxin is disastrous and non-homœopathic.

Study in this connection:

The Organon: The Introduction, called by Hahnemann, "A Review of Therapeutics; allopathy and palliative treatment, that have hitherto been practiced in the old-school of medicine," together with historical intimations of Homœopathy before Hahnemann's time.

Also, Organon § 1-6, on the Functions of the Physician.

Also, Homœopathy, the Science of Therapeutics, by Carroll Dunham.

Homœopathy, the only system of curative medicine, by Charles S. Mack.

Pathogenic Therapeutics, by J. P. Dake, in his Therapeutic Methods.

Hahnemann's criticism of Isopathy, in the Organon, Introduction, note 34.

Dr. Dudgeon's most valuable appendix to his translation and edition of the Organon, page 200.

CHAPTER II.

PRINCIPLES OF PHARMACOLOGY.

Pharmacology (*pharmakon*, a drug, *logos* a discourse) is a convenient term for the whole subject of Materia Medica, pharmacy and medicinal therapeutics. Specifically, it refers often to drug effects, as evinced from experiments on animals, and as such is the only source of modern old-school knowledge of the physiological action of drugs.

Materia Medica is the study of drugs in regard to their origin, physical and chemical properties, but especially and chiefly in regard to their effects in modifying the health of the body. The latter is the distinctive field of the Homœopathic Materia Medica.

Drugs and Drug Action. Drugs are substances taken from all the kingdoms of nature that are used as medicines. They usually produce deleterious effects upon the body when given in sufficiently large doses in health, and they modify some part, or the whole, of a morbid state when given to the sick. This property is discovered either empirically by observation of cases of poisoning, or by systematic experiments on human beings in health.

Medicinal force is a distinct property of drugs, by which they modify vital activity, not by their chemical, physical or mechanical properties, but by their specific dynamic property, peculiar, distinctive and different in every drug. And they can be truly *curative* only by reason of their modifying properties of the vital processes. Each medicinal substance, be it plant, mineral or animal product, has stored within its material particles, and embodies, therefore, its own particular medicinal force, which can be brought into activity by breaking up the outward particles. The character of this specific force, or the drug's medicinal properties, can only be discovered by the vital test, made by experimenting with different doses on healthy human organisms, and to some extent on animals. The latter merely to see the ultimate lesions and organic changes drugs are able to produce.

At one time, and especially during the middle ages, before the introduction of modern, scientific methods, the properties of drugs were based upon the

Doctrine of Signatures. External characteristics of a substance served to indicate possible therapeutic effects. Fancied or real resemblances between some part of a plant and some particular organ or fluid of the body pointed to therapeutic relationship. Thus, according to this doctrine, Digitalis must be of use in blood diseases, because its flowers are adorned with blood colored dots; Euphrasia was famous as a remedy for the eyes, because it had a black spot in its coralla, which looked like a pupil.*

The lungs of a fox must be specific against asthma, because this animal has a very vigorous respiration.

Hypericum having red juice ought therefore to be of use in hæmorrhages.

Euphorbia, having a milky juice, must be good for increasing the flow of milk.

Sticta, having some likeness to the lungs, was called pulmonarius and esteemed as a remedy for pulmonary complaints.

Singularly enough, in isolated instances at least, such relationship actually does exist, as has been verified by subsequent clinical application, and it is possible that an intuitively gifted race may see a relationship actu-

* Grauvogl.

ally existing between outward forms and structures and inner uses. But for purposes of modern scientific therapeutics it is valueless.*

Other methods of determining the medicinal virtues of drugs were by the sense of taste and of smell. Drugs with a bitter taste were held to possess tonic and stomachic virtues, hence the "Bitters" of the ordinary pharmacopœia. Gentiana, for instance, is such a drug, and unquestionably does exert a tonic influence upon the stomach. But this virtue is probably not because it is bitter, but because it has a distinctive medicinal force wholly independent of its taste. Certain aromatic drugs were deemed to possess anti-spasmodic and stimulant properties, etc.

Experimental Pharmacology. The modern method for arriving at a knowledge of drugs is by experimentation on animals, chiefly frogs, rabbits, dogs, cats, etc. But this method is objectionable on account of the difference in structure and physiology of these animals

---

* "The soul does not perceive the external or internal physical construction of herbs and roots, but it intuitively perceives their powers and virtues and recognizes at once their *signatum*. This signature is a certain organic vital activity giving each natural object (in contra-distinction to artificially made objects) a certain similarity with a certain condition produced by disease, and through which health may be restored in specific diseases in the diseased part. This signatum is often expressed, even in the exterior form of things, and by observing that form we may learn something in regard to their interior qualities, even without using our interior sight. We see that the internal character of a man is often expressed in his exterior appearance, even in the manner of his walking, and in the sound of his voice. Likewise the hidden character of things is to a certain extent expressed in their outward forms. As long as man remained in a natural state, he recognized the signatures of things and knew their true character; but the more he diverged from the path of nature and the more his mind became captivated by illusive external appearances, the more this power became lost."—*Paracelsus.*

and the vast difference in their susceptibility to the action of medicines. Nux is most poisonous to man, yet pigs can eat it freely; Aconite is fatal to man in a small dose, yet dogs and horses can eat it with impunity. Birds are not susceptible to the action of Opium or Atropin, etc. Again, the dynamic effects of drugs differ among animals. For instance, Ipecac and Tartar Emetic are emetics to men and dogs, but not to rabbits. Such methods of arriving at the crude drug effects may be sufficient to determine the so-called physiological effects of drugs, and the antipathic use of them based thereon, but is wholly inadequate for purposes of Homœopathy. They have their use, also, in determining the ultimate organic lesions produced by certain drugs, whenever it is desirable to push a proving to such an extent.

Physiological action of drugs. Drugs produce in the organism, when given in sufficiently large doses, certain disturbances or alterations of function, usually of a correspondingly definite character. The dosage required for this purpose is, as a rule, a fixed one within certain limits. It is the *physiological dose*—that is, a dose large enough to *produce* symptoms. Opium constipates the bowels, produces insensibility. For these purposes a recognized, fixed quantity is necessary, not less than one-half to one grain. This constitutes its physiological dose. Strychnia increases the reflex excitability of the spinal cord, in doses of one-twelfth to one-thirtieth of a grain. Digitalis slows the heart in ten minim doses.

Now this direct, absolute action of drugs, which is constant, can be made the basis of treatment of disease, wherever this is possible. Its advantages are immediate results and improvement of certain conditions opposed to this direct drug action. It is, therefore, palliative where indicated. This use of drugs is based upon the law of *contraria contrariis opponenda*, when an opposite result is desired, or when it is intended to produce not an opposite, but an entirely different action, as, for instance, a purgative in a case of headache. The objections to this direct use of drug effects, by means of physiological dosage, are the limited field to which such action is applicable and the necessity for increasing dosage, and sooner or later opposite reactionary results that make further use of the drug useless. All physicians may make use of this direct, physiological action of certain drugs for certain conditions, but its usefulness is limited. Hahnemann himself clearly defines it as follows:

"I do not fail to recognize the great ability of palliatives. They are often not only quite sufficient in cases appearing suddenly and developing rapidly, but they have great advantages, indeed, where aid cannot be postponed for an hour, or even a minute. Here, and here alone, are palliatives of real use."

This use of drugs for their *direct* primary effects by means of a dosage sufficiently large and within certain limits, always definite and precise, has led to a classification of drugs, according to their physiological and some of their therapeutic actions, and not differing materially from that introduced by Dioscorides, the father of Materia Medica. Since his time drugs have been classified into three principal classes, evacuants, alteratives and specifics. The evacuants are again subdivided with respect to the various routes by which nature expels the morbid matters, such as purgatives, expectorants and diaphoretics. Alteratives comprise drugs which alter the course of morbid conditions, modifying the nutritive processes while promoting waste, and thus indirectly curing some chronic diseases;

such are Mercury, Iodine and Arsenic. *They increase metabolism.*

Other classes are the antipyretics, emmenagogues, styptics, anthelmintics, astringents, etc., etc.

While such classification is very imperfect, and but a partial designation of the properties of drugs, for every drug may belong to several classes, and its special properties in any class are at best vague and uncertain, still, there is some advantage to those who want to avail themselves of the direct drug effects, of this drug classification, based on some of their more marked pathogenetic and therapeutic effects. *But it is entirely useless for homœopathic prescribing.*

The homœopathic method by means of drug experimentation on the healthy, so-called drug proving. This is the only scientific and rational method of ascertaining the action of medicines. All other methods have proved useless and misleading. The credit of first teaching the necessity of proving drugs upon the healthy belongs to Albrecht von Haller, a Swiss physician. As early as 1755, in his Swiss pharmacopœia, he distinctly taught this, but nothing came of it. It was not until Samuel Hahnemann, in 1796, practically went to work and actually experimented with drugs on himself and others that the first pure effects of drugs became known and could be rationally employed in practice. Hahnemann was thus the founder of the science of drug pathogenesy, for it is a fact that up to his time no one had made any physiological experiment with any drug; it is a fact that his experiments with Peruvian Bark were the first ever made in the domain of pharmacology, and are a model to this day. The science of drug proving dates therefore from 1796, and is the beginning of a rational therapeutics. With the adoption of this principle, we have a key to unlock the sphere of action of every substance in nature, so far as it can bear any relation to man's constitution in health and disease. It is a creative principle, universal in its application, true for all time. The introduction of in into medicine marks an epoch in the development o the healing art, before which time a science of thera peutics was impossible.

In the Organon, §§ 108–9, Hahnemann says:

"There is, therefore, no other possible way in which the peculiar effects of medicine on the health of indi viduals can be accurately ascertained; there is no sure no more natural way of accomplishing this object that to administer the several medicines experimentally, if moderate doses, to *healthy* persons, in order to ascer tain what changes, symptoms and signs of their influ ence each individual produces on the health of th body and of the mind; that is to say, what disease ele ments they are able and tend to produce, since, as ha been demonstrated, all the curative power of medi cines lies in the power they possess of changing th state of man's health, and is revealed by observation o the latter."

Drug Pathogenesy is the record of testing drugs on the human body in varying doses, and on differen individuals of both sexes, and observing all the symp toms, subjective and objective, from the minutest dis turbed function and mental state to the grossest organi lesion. "Simple drugs," says Hahnemann, "produce in the healthy body symptoms peculiar to themselves but not all at once, nor in one and the same series, no all in each experimenter." Such a method of arrivin at a knowledge of drugs is universal in its application it includes all that can be learned from toxicology alsc

The value of toxicology as illustrating drug action is far inferior, however, to that of testing them in health by means of small doses. Still it gives the ultimate lesions and organic changes, and in this way interprets many symptoms of the provings; but whenever the organism is violently invaded by a foreign destructive agent, no matter what the poison is, there is usually much similarity of action, resulting from nature's efforts to throw it off by all possible routes outward from the body's distinctive vital centers, hence the inevitable nausea, vomiting, diarrhœa, nerve disturbances, convulsions, paralysis, etc., of most poisonings. The provings with small doses avoid these crude, extreme effects, and, instead of producing them, rather indicate them by the milder disturbances produced.

Different Applications of Drug-action. The knowledge of what drugs will do when given to a healthy subject can be utilized in two different ways, both legitimate, and it is a mere matter of experience and observation to determine which is the better. We can use a drug to *produce* its physiological effects. If this is desired, the drug must be given in a dose large enough to produce symptoms—that is, in a so-called physiological dose, differing with each drug and determined by experiment. This is the antipathic use of drugs, and *has nothing to do with Homœopathy*, or the law of cure. It is, moreover, very limited in its application, and objectionable on many grounds.

The other method, the homœopathic relationship, is universal in its application, and is not confined to any special dosage, provided such always is sub-physiological—*i. e., less* than is required to *produce* symptoms. Hence, *drugs can act in two different ways when given in disease,* and we can have, therefore:

1. Homœopathic relationship—when given for conditions similar to those they are capable of producing. Applicable to all drugs, and universal in its extent.

(2) Antipathic or allopathic relationship—when given in physiological dosage to produce their first, direct or physiological effects. This is, as we have stated before, of but very limited application.

The only difference in the application of drugs to disease with the two schools of medicine is, that the old school gives drugs solely to obtain their direct, physiological effects, and rather favors combination of remedies, while the homœopathic school depends entirely upon the curative results obtained by giving the single remedy in a sub-physiological dose for symptoms similar to those it is known to produce.

For reference and further study, see Hahnemann's Essay on a New Principle for Ascertaining the Curative Powers of Drugs in his Lesser Writings, page 249.

Hahnemann's Essay on the Sources of the Common Materia Medica, being Preface to Vol. II of the Materia Medica Pura.

The Physiological Action of Medicines, by Wm. Sharp, in Essays on Medicine, page 417.

General Principles of Drug Action, by R. Hughes, in Pharmacodynamics; lecture IV-V.

An interesting account and practical application of the Doctrine of Signatures can be found in Grauvogl's Textbook, § 91-95.

Samuel A Jones, M.D.: "The Grounds of a Homœopath's Faith." An inspiring little work.

Dudgeon. "Lectures on Homœopathy." Lect. VI, Isopathy.

CHAPTER III.

THE EVOLUTION OF THE HOMŒOPATHIC MATERIA MEDICA.

The Homœopathic Materia Medica is a record of the effects of drugs upon the healthy human organism, embodying a knowledge of what drugs actually do when brought in contact with the functional activity of the body. The sources of this knowledge are,

1. The systematic provings.
2. Observations of cases of poisoning and over-dosings, which Hahnemann and his disciples have gathered from general medical literature.

The First Book on Drug Effects. The first work embodying such record is that of Hahnemann, entitled *Fragmenta de Viribus Medicamentorum Positivis.* It is a Latin work, and published in Leipsic in 1805. Twenty-seven drugs are treated of, containing symptoms Hahnemann himself had observed as effects of poisoning or from excessive dosing, and of provings on himself.* "I have instituted experiments," he says in the preface, " in chief part on my own person, but also on some others whom I knew to be perfectly healthy and free from all perceptible disease."

"In those experiments which have been made by myself and my disciples, every care has been taken to

* It is interesting to know the names of the pioneer medicines whose pathogenic effects were first published in this work of Hahnemann. They are Aconitum, Arnica, Belladonna, Camphora, Cantharis, Capsicum, Causticum, Chamomilla, Cinchona, Cocculus, Copaiva, Cuprum, Digitalis, Drosera, Helleborus, Hyoscyamus, Ignatia, Ipecacuanha, Ledum, Mezereum, Nux vomica, Opium, Pulsatilla, Rheum, Stramonium, Valeriana, Veratrum album. Of these, Cantharis, Copaiva, and Valeriana, Hahnemann did not include in his subsequently published "Materia Medica."

secure the true and full action of the medicines. Our provings have been made upon persons in perfect health, and living in contentment and comparative ease. When an extraordinary circumstance of any kind—fright, chagrin, external injuries, the excessive enjoyment of any one pleasure, or some event of great importance—supervened during the proving, then no other symptom has been recorded after such an event, in order to prevent spurious symptoms being noted as genuine. When such circumstances were of slight importance, and could hardly be supposed to interfere with the action of the medicine, the symptoms have been placed in brackets, for the purpose of informing the reader that they could not be considered decisively genuine."

Hahnemann's Materia Medica Pura.

Five years now elapsed before Hahnemann published anything more in the line of drug pathogenesy. They must have been five years of intense labor and experiment. Then appeared the first volume of that great classical work, the "Materia Medica Pura," containing the symptomatology of twelve medicines, six of which had already appeared in the Latin treatise published before.

Five years later appeared the second volume, containing the symptomatology of eight medicines, which was soon succeeded by the four other volumes, containing in all the pathogenic effects of sixty-one drugs. It is a monumental work, the result of Hahnemann's matchless penetration, wonderful insight and accurate observation, of which he was a master. He was most ably assisted in this work by thirty-five fellow-provers, among whom the names of Franz, Gross, Hartmann, Herrmann, Hornburg, Rückert, Stapf, and Friedrich Hahnemann are the most conspicuous and deserve to be remembered by all students of Materia Medica.

In 1822 appeared a second edition of this great work, with considerable additions to the symptomatology of all the remedies and some new medicines besides. A third and fourth edition were published after some years.

Publication of the "Chronic Diseases."

In 1828 Hahnemann published his "Chronic Diseases," containing the symptomatology of a completely new series of medicines, a series of deeply-acting drugs, like Calcarea, Sulphur, etc., the so-called Anti-psoric remedies. The symptomatology of these remedies was not wholly pathogenetic, but included observations at the bedside, so-called clinical symptoms.

A second edition, greatly enlarged and now containing the symptomatology of twenty-five remedies, besides the twenty-two of the first edition, appeared between 1835 and 1839. A peculiar feature of the provings in this work is that the bulk of them must have been obtained with the thirtieth potency, and often are observations when given to the sick, differing entirely, therefore, from the pathogenetic effects of the Materia Medica Pura. A new English translation of this great work has just appeared in this country.

Besides Hahnemann and his immediate disciples, Constantine Hering, of Philadelphia, contributed the best provings to the homœopathic Materia Medica, some of his drugs ranking in importance with Hahnemann's own. Of these, Lachesis, Glonoine and Apis take first rank.

Another large contributor to the Materia Medica was Dr. E. M. Hale, not so much by proving as by introducing American remedies that had been in use by botanic physicians, and gathering all that was known as to the therapeutic properties in one volume, called "New Remedies." We have, then, as

Sources of the Homœopathic Materia Medica.

1. Hahnemann's Materia Medica Pura, published in 1811, containing the pathogenesis of the great polychrests—*i. e.*, remedies of many uses and wide and frequent application.

2. Hahnemann's Chronic Diseases, published in 1828, containing the so-called Antipsoric remedies, those especially adapted to the cure of chronic diseases.

3. Dr. Jörg's Provings—a professor at the University of Leipsic and contemporary of Hahnemann, but not one of his followers. He proved, among others, Camphor, Digitalis, Opium, Arnica, Hydrocy. acid, Ignatia. Some of his symptoms are quoted and included by Hahnemann in the second edition of his works.

4. Dr. Hering and the American Provers' Union.

5. Dr. E. M. Hale's contributions in his "New Remedies."

6. Various provings and reprovings under the auspices of the American Institute of Homœopathy, various State societies and individual provings published in our journalistic literature. Also, Hartlaub and Trink's pathogeneses, Stapf's additions, provings by the Austrian Society, etc., etc.

These records are at present collected in three great works:

1. "Allen's Enclycopædia," in ten volumes.

2. "Cyclopædia of Drug Pathogenesy," in four volumes.

These two works contain the symptoms obtained by provings, and from records of poisoning, *i. e.*, *pathogenetic symptoms.*

3. "Hering's Guiding Symptoms," in ten volumes, which *also contains clinical or curative symptoms*—*i. e.*, observed on the sick.

The comparative value of the three sources of symptoms, from records of toxicology, provings on healthy and observation on sick.

1. *Toxicology.* Violent cases of poisoning never yield a profitable symptomatology, on account of the violent invasion by foreign destructive agents. The organism throws it off by all routes outward and away from its distinctive life, hence vomiting, diarrhœa, convulsions, etc., common to all kinds of poisoning. On the other hand, the records of poisoning give us the ultimate action, the tissue and organic changes that the provings can only indicate, and thus they illustrate and interpret the provings.

2. *Provings on the healthy.* The provings with comparatively small doses avoid these violent, crude and extreme effects, and instead of producing them, rather indicate them by mild disturbances. We thus obtain the finer and more characteristic action, and thus a much more utilizable picture of drug effects. Fortunately, the bulk of the homœopathic Materia Medica is made up from this source. The symptoms obtained from toxicological observations and from provings are also called *pathogenetic symptoms,* and the full record, in the order of their development, is called the drug's *pathogenesis.* The "Cyclopædia of Drug Pathogenesy" gives these in their fullest and most accurate form.

3. *Drug effects observed in the sick.* In the evolution of the homœopathic Materia Medica, another class of symptoms not bearing the aristocracy of origin, characterizing pathogenetic symptoms, were introduced, so-called *clinical or curative symptoms.* This source was almost unavoidable, so long as drug provings on the healthy were limited in number and extent. The symptomatology of most of the great constitutional or anti-psoric remedies consists, in large part, of such clin-

ical symptoms. They are such symptoms as disappear after administering a remedy, and which are not found among the pathogenetic effects, so far as the provings have been made; but, wherever genuine, there can be no doubt that they are *possible* pathogenetic symptoms, could we have full and accurate provings. In this way the homœopathic Materia Medica has been enlarged, not always wisely, however; for, in order to discover them amidst the symptoms of the disease in a patient, much discrimination and training are required. Hahnemann rightly says that this is a "subject for the exercise of a higher order of inductive minds, and must be left solely to masters in the art of observation." But, when found, they must be used tentatively and cautiously until verified in practice. Only then can they be admitted by the side of the true pathogenetic symptoms and form a legitimate addition to the Materia Medica. Some of the greatest characteristics and guiding symptoms belong to this class. These clinical symptoms have been excluded from the "Encyclopædia of Materia Medica" by T. F. Allen, and, of course, cannot have any place in the "Cyclopædia of Drug Pathogenesy"; but they are included in full in Hering's "Guiding Symptoms" and in all manuals and text-books of Materia Medica. In some of these they are designated by a distinguishing mark, usually O, but in most of the later works even this caution is disregarded.

The Hahnemannian Schema. In order to bring this vast symptomatology within the ready reference of the busy practitioner, Hahnemann, himself a physician of large and extensive practice, and, hence, in need of labor-saving devices, re-arranged it in anatomical order, which has been found so practical for every-day use, that it has been universally adopted by all our authors on Materia Medica. He begins with the head and first records all the symptoms of the mind, sensorium, etc.; then those of the eyes, nose, face, etc., downwards, placing together all the symptoms relating to each section. In this way the original provings were dissected, destroying the order of development of the symptoms, but greatly facilitating ready reference.

The Repertory or Index of Symptoms. This is another aid that has been found necessary to facilitate the selection of the indicated remedy. It is a useful appendage to the homœopathic Materia Medica, by means of which we can readily discover almost any recorded symptom of any proven drug. The secret of successful use of the "Repertory" is to get thoroughly acquainted with any one of the different repertories by constant reference to it, thus familiarizing oneself with its peculiar arrangement. The most helpful of them all, but the one requiring, also, most patient study, is Boeninghausen's "Therapeutic Pocket Book." Its arrangement is based on a practical analysis of symptoms into their component elements of location, sensation and conditions. (See Chapter V.)

How to learn Drug Pathogenesy and acquire a working knowledge of the homœopathic Materia Medica has occupied the students of Homœopathy from the beginning of the school. Unquestionably, the proving of a drug is the truly natural and most effective method of getting a knowledge of its action, and every physician and student should undertake such practical study as at least part of his study of materia medica. It is the true, modern, scientific method by appeal to nature herself. In the absence of this, and as a further aid, the study of original provings, and of records of poisonings, will go far to give a good general outline of the action of a drug. This should be followed by the careful and repeated reading of the recorded symptomatology, noting the *parts* especially involved, *character* of the symptoms, the *conditions* under which they occur, and the *concomitants* connected with each symptom. In this way the peculiar and characteristic symptoms and conditions will appear, which will be the guiding symptoms in practice. These characteristics, so-called key-notes, of the different remedies, must be committed to memory, they form the stock in trade of the homœopathic prescriber, and will lead to the further and more detailed and comparative study of the remedies.

For further study, consult Hughes, "Sources of the Homœopathic Materia Medica," in his work on Pharmacodynamics; also published separately by Leath & Ross, London.

Dr. John W. Hayward: "How to Learn Drug Pathogenesy," with discussion, in the *Journal of the British Homœopathic Society*, January, 1895.

The following classical papers should also be consulted:

Constantine Hering: "How the Materia Medica should be Learnt," in *British Journal of Homœopathy*, Vol. II.

Dr. Meyer, one of Hahnemann's immediate disciples, on the same subject, in *North American Journal of Homœopathy*, Vol. II.

Dr. Pope, in *Monthly Homœopathic Review*, VIII, and Vol. XXV.

Dr. H. R. Madden, in same journal, Vol. XIV.

Dr. R. Hughes, in same journal, Vol. XXIII, and in *Hahnemannian Monthly*, Vol. XXIX.

Dr. C. Wesselhoeft in *N. E. Medical Gazette*, Vol. XXII.

Dr. Joseph C. Guernsey, in *Hahnemannian Monthly*, Vol. XXIX.

American Institute Report for 1894, Materia Medica Section; opinions of thirty-one members. Edited by Dr. Frank Kraft.

CHAPTER IV.

DRUG PROVING.

The proving of medicines is a distinctive feature of Homœopathy and a logical necessity for applying the law of cure; for, in order to meet morbid states with drugs corresponding to them, we must know, and therefore ascertain, what morbid states the different medicinal substances produce. It consists in the systematic testing of a drug on the healthy human body, in order to ascertain the changes which it is capable of producing in the functions and organs.

Hahnemann, after viewing the subject in every possible light, and examining every method for ascertaining the action of drugs, came to the conclusion that the only efficient way was "to test the medicines singly and alone on the healthy human body."

General Rules for Drug Proving. The medicinal substance which is to be proved must be tested singly, without any admixture of any foreign substance, except an inert vehicle when necessary for its administration. Nothing of a medicinal nature should be taken so long as it is desired to observe the effects of the proving.

Each drug should be proved, not only in its crude form and lower material dosage, but with higher attenuations as well. When the latter are used and symptoms obtained, a special susceptibility on the part of the prover probably exists and some of the most important characteristics may be elicited from him. Only actually observed facts should be recorded, free from all theories of drug action. Such purely positive observation is for all time, and possesses the same value after the lapse of centuries as it does at the time when first observed. If any deductions be drawn from the observed facts, they should not be incorporated into the text, but kept separate and distinct. For this reason, Hahnemann called his Materia Medica "Pura" (pure), because free from all theories, only a record of observed facts. Hence, in making a proving, great precaution, control experiment, accuracy, close observation, and the strictest conscientiousness are essential.

Directions for provers. The prover should not depart in any material way from any of his ordinary habits of life, because his life is based on these habits and conformed to them, and any marked change in these must result in changes more or less important, which might be put to the account of the drug; hence, his food, drink, sleep, exercise, and habits generally must be such as he has been accustomed to. He should observe himself before beginning a proving, as every one is liable, even in the best state of health, to slight variations in his sensations and functions. Having thus discovered what symptoms he is liable to naturally and without any drug influence, he must avoid attributing these to the drug to be proven, unless, indeed, they are more pronounced than ever.

Dosage required for proving. As a general rule, begin with a comparatively small dose and increase it gradually till distinct symptoms make their appearance. The most useful doses are those that are just sufficient to produce distinct symptoms.

Female provers. It is very important to test all drugs in regard to their effects on the female organism, hence women, married and unmarried, should contribute to provings. "Before beginning the record of a proving, she should inscribe in the note-book a statement of her age, temperament, the sicknesses which she has had, and those to which she has an inherited or acquired tendency; also, whatever pains or sensations she may be habitually subject to; also, any peculiar susceptibilities she may possess to external influences of any kind, or to mental, or moral, or emotional excitements, depressions or perversions. Her constitutional peculiarities, respecting the menstrual function, should be carefully recorded; regarding frequency, quantity, character, and whatever inconveniences or sufferings precede, accompany or follow menstruation, such as headache, backache, colic, leucorrhœa, etc., with peculiar states of mind or emotion." *

Repetition of doses. No special rule can be given, but it has been the custom of most provers to repeat the dose every few hours until symptoms show themselves. It is best to give a single, rather large, dose and watch its effects. This plan is chiefly useful with some vegetable medicines, whose sphere of action is small, and of which the first dose sometimes exhausts, for a time, the susceptibility of the system to the action of the substance. The continuous repetition of the dose is applicable, if we want to ascertain the special action of a drug on some organ or function by continued dosing.

Age and sex are modifying factors in drug proving, and all drugs should be tried on individuals of both sexes and different ages. Some drugs possess marked affinity for one sex, as Crocus and Platina for the female, and Nux preferably the male.

Temperament. Different temperaments should be chosen, for certain medicines are especially adapted to certain temperaments, and here find the most favorable environment for developing their specific effects.

---

* Dunham.

Re-provings. The provings should be repeated in different individuals and in the same prover. In order to avoid the admission of accidental symptoms, it is a safe rule, although not absolute, not to adopt any symptoms unless it has been found in several provers. By comparing one proving with another, and ascertaining the constancy with which the different symptoms appear, the characteristic symptoms are made manifest. It is to be remembered that all individuals are not alike susceptible to all the effects which a drug is capable of producing; therefore, the need of a large number of experiments is apparent, in order to obtain a complete view of the action of a drug.

Hering's Rules for Provers.

(1) Make a first experimental test with a single, moderate-sized dose.

(2) If no symptoms are produced, take it every two or three hours, or change the time of the day for taking it.

(3) If still no symptoms, try higher potencies, to which might be added this rational, additional rule: if still no symptoms appear, go lower in the scale of attenuations and give material doses, increasing size until symptoms appear.

In the nature of things, some of the symptoms take time to develop, therefore the first experiments with small doses should not be hurried. The prover should learn to wait, for some of the late appearing symptoms are frequently the most characteristic.

How to Describe Symptoms Obtained from a Proving. The greatest minuteness and accuracy should be observed. A sensation should be described by some familiar comparison. State how the symptom is effected by different circumstances, i. e., the drug's modalities, as position of body, motion, rest, eating, fasting, day, night, indoors, open air, weather, etc. No circumstance, however trifling, should be omitted which may in any way tend to indicate the characteristic action of the drug and so precisionize it. All such conditions of aggravation and amelioration should be carefully recorded as they express the drug's individuality most clearly and universally.

The *sides* of the body on which symptoms occur should always be stated, many remedies acting more markedly on one side than another.

The *times* of occurence, aggravation or amelioration, are also very important, some remedies having distinctive morning aggravation of some or all of their symptoms, others at night, etc. As an illustration of a perfect description of a symptom, take the following of Hahnemann's proving of Nux: " Headache beginning some hours before dinner, increased after eating, then violent shooting pain in left temple, with nausea and very acid vomiting, all of which symptoms disappeared on lying down."

The three essential features of every complete symptom are, therefore,

(1) Location.

(2) Sensation.

(3) Condition of aggravation or amelioration (modality), which is the most important, and it ought to be the aim of all provers to observe symptoms with these features well in mind.

Never separate symptoms that appear in groups or with marked concomitants. Hahnemann always left together symptoms appearing in groups, if he considered them really connected; for instance, he observed, forty-five minutes after taking Pulsatilla, a cramp in the legs, in the evening, after lying down, with a chill; and at another time, in the evening, an aching, drawing pain in the legs up into the knee, with more chilliness than during the day.

Primary and Secondary Drug Effects. It is a law of drug action, according to which the administration of each medicine causes, at first, certain abnormal symptoms, the so-called *primary* effects of medicines, but afterwards, by reaction of the organism, a condition entirely the opposite, where this is possible, of this first effect is produced—the *secondary* effects, for instance, narcotic substances produce primarily insensibility and secondarily pain. In order to produce the *primary* effects, material doses are required.

In his essay, entitled "Suggestions for Ascertaining the Curative Powers of Drugs," Hahnemann says: "Most medicines have more than one action; the first a direct action, which gradually changes into the second (which I call the indirectly secondary action). The latter is generally a state exactly the opposite of the former. In this way most vegetable drugs act. But few medicines are exceptions to this rule, *i. e.*, metals and minerals. The thorough examination of drug provings, as in our possession at present, does not justify any division of drug-symptoms into primary and secondary. There are indeed in every proving, as Dr. Hering has shown, primary and secondary symptoms, *in the sense that some symptoms appear earlier and others later in the course of the proving*, but although these may appear opposed to each other, they are all to be regarded as drug symptoms, and, as such, indicate the remedy.

Hahnemann's method of conducting provings. Dr. Hering thus describes it: "After he had lectured to his fellow-workers on the rules of proving, he handed them the bottles with the tincture; and when they afterwards brought him their day books, he examined every prover carefully about every particular symptom, continually calling attention to the necessary accuracy in expressing the kind of feeling, the pain or the locality, the observation and mentioning of everything that influenced their feelings, the time of day, etc. When handing their papers to him, after they had been cross-examined, they had to affirm that it was the truth, and nothing but the truth, to the best of their knowledge, by offering their hands to him—the customary pledge at the universities of Germany, instead of an oath. This was the way in which our master built up his Materia Medica."

For fuller study see Organon, § 105 to 145.

Dudgeon, Lectures on Homœopathy, page 176. Lecture VII and VIII.

Sharp's Tracts on Homœopathy, Essay VII. Provings in Health.

Dunham, Science of Therapeutics: The Dose in Drug Proving, page 136. Directions for Drug Provers, page 350.

CHAPTER V.

INTERPRETATION OF DRUG PATHOGENESIS.

The homœopathic Matèria Medica, as it is accessible at present to students, is a mass of symptomatology, arranged, as a rule, according to the Hahnemannian Schema. The "Cyclopædia of Drug Pathogenesy" is the exception, which endeavors to give the symptoms in the order of their development; but, in order to practically utilize the provings, the anatomical arrangement of the symptomatology is desirable. Besides this arrangement, the bulk of the symptomatology can be analyzed and interpreted helpfully, and thus simplified. All provings of drugs give a symptomatology composed

(1) Of general symptoms.

(2) Of peculiar or characteristic symptoms.

(3) Of certain elective affinities to special organs or functions.

General symptoms of drugs. These are common to all drugs and appear in every proving. They can practically be eliminated. Such are symptoms like feeling of malaise, loss of appetite, weakness, distress, headache, etc. Such general symptoms, *unless amplified by accompanying conditions or modalities*, are of comparatively little value for the prescriber, because their presence does not point clearly to any one particular drug. We must find in our symptomatology, and make use of such symptoms as serve to individualize and give character to a drug, and hence these are called

Characteristic Symptoms. Each drug is an entity, and can express its disease producing properties, *i. e.*, pathogenetic force, in a way peculiar to itself. Those symptoms that do this most perfectly are the drug's characteristic symptoms. The ideal characteristic symptom is one which is possessed by no other than the individual drug of which it is predicated and to which it gives character as an individual. We learn to distinguish drugs very much as we learn to distinguish men, not by their general features, which are common to all, but rather by the peculiar expression and shape and habits by which we recognize the individual. It may be a small and insignificant thing and yet one that is most expressive of the person's individuality. So in drugs it is not the general effect upon the stomach or bowels or the general debility produced that serve to characterize it as the remedy, but rather the *peculiar*, characteristic uncommon, prominent symptoms.

These have also been designated as *keynote* * *symptoms*, by Dr. Guernsey, and as *guiding symptoms*, by Dr. Hering.

From a physiological point of view they may appear trivial and unimportant, but for purposes of prescribing they are paramount in importance. These characteristic symptoms of drugs may be found in one of three divisions of its pathogenesis. Either

---

* "While the *keynotes*, according to Dr. Guernsey, will, in each instance, form an unfailing guide, the requisite conditions and corresponding totality of the symptoms in such cases being inevitably present. If this doctrine is true—and in practice it has been confirmed by much experience—it is so because these so-called *keynotes* essentially represent a profound dyscrasia of the *organic nervous system*; either in such sensations of pain as precede even the first functional derangements, and are intended as premonitory admonitions; or in such sensations as arise in connection with, and in consequence of, the initial disorder in these most interior organs of vegetative life."—*J. H. P. Frost in Hahnemannian Monthly, Vol. II, page* 443.

1. In the locality or tissue or organ affected.
2. In the sensations.
3. In the modalities and concomitants.

These are the three grand divisions around which the symptomatology of drugs can be grouped, or into which they can be divided for practical study.

Locality or seat of action. Every drug affects some organ or system of organs or tissue or region more decidedly than others, and there especially or primarily expends its power. This is not a local action merely, but *a localization of the drug's specific nature.* It appears, no matter by what avenue the drug is introduced into the body. A drug may come into direct contact with the blood, and thereby with every part of the organism, and yet only certain tissues or organs will be affected by it—that is, only these tissues or organs will react against the foreign element. This specific localization, or specificity of seat of a drug, is known as its *elective affinity*, by which it preferably chooses certain cells, tissues or organs, to manifest its action. In a general way, we see that Belladonna affects principally the brain as its arena for action, and this organ, therefore, has a preferred relationship to Belladonna. So, in the same way, Aconite affects the heart, Ergot the uterus, Bryonia the serous membranes, Podophyllum the duodenum, Rhus the skin; Tellurium, the tympanum; Glonoin the vaso-motor centre in the brain; Phosphor. the periosteum.

This elective affinity cannot be explained, but it exists. It was recognized even before Hahnemann and homœopathic provings, and has been made the foundation of a system of practice by Rademacher, a German physician and contemporary of Hahnemann, who himself traces the thought to Paracelsus.

While each drug has a preferred locality, based on

its elective affinity, still it must not be forgotten that the whole organism—the whole man, mentally and physically,—is affected. This is so, because the various functions and organs are not independent instruments, but wonderfully bound together by nerves and blood vessels, and parts most remote are in direct nerve communication with each other. Diseases are produced and continued along these lines of network, when once they have found a foothold, and drugs act in a similar manner along these tracks. We ought to get a mental picture of a drug as a whole—the drug personified, and thus the typical patient corresponding to the drug. Such study gives a reality and practical utility to the Materia Medica.

Sensations, or kind of Action. While the special *seat* of action is the first marked fact about the pathogenetic properties of drugs, the special *kind* of action is the second fact. This may be seen in the sensations and modalities of a drug. Thus the *burning* pains of Arsenic, the *coldness* of Camphor and Veratrum, the *sticking* pains of Bryonia, the *stinging* pains of Apis and Theridion, the plug sensations of Anacardium, the *soreness* of Arnica and Hamamelis, are all characteristic. Frequently the character of these pains indicates the *seat* of the action, and thus points to the elective affinity of the drug, as burning pains in general indicate the mucous membranes; dull, boring, gnawing pains, the bones; sticking, cutting pains, serous membranes; etc. In many drugs these conditions may be so expressive of their special character, that we nearly always expect them to be present when they are the homœopathically indicated, and, therefore, prove to be the curative remedy. Such characteristic conditions are the restlessness and anxiety of Aconite and Arsenic, the chilliness of Pulsatilla, the thirstlessness of Apis, the dullness and drowsiness of Gelsemium, the hysterial contradiction of its symptoms of Ignatia, the melancholy of Aurum, etc.

Modalities and Concomitants. Modalities are conditions influencing or modifying drug action. They are the phenomena of time, place, circumstances on which the development and appearance of the symptoms depend. Every drug has its own mode of action, manifests itself in a way peculiar to itself, distinguishing it from every other. It acts best under certain conditions, in certain bodily and mental constitutions, which present, therefore, the most favorable ground and environment for the full and free manifestation of the drug's individuality. Just as a plant thrives best in certain conditions of soil, climate, elevation, etc.—needs, in short, for its perfect development, a suitable environment,—so a drug must be similarly situated to enable it to express itself clearly and fully. It is of the greatest importance in drug proving, as well as in prescribing homœopathically, to note the peculiar method in which a drug invades the animal economy, its aggravations and ameliorations, the times of the day, and conditions of the weather, when the action is most pronounced. For instance, the marked increase of pain on motion of Bryonia, the relief of headache by wrapping head up warmly of Silica, the marked preference of the left side of the body of Lachesis, the aggravation of all the symptoms from 4 to 8 P. M. of Lycopodium, the relief by heat of Arsenic, the aggravation of damp weather of Dulcamara, are characteristic conditions of great value, clearly expressing the peculiar genius of these drugs and are paramount in estimating their place in the symptomatology. But, while they hold this important place, they must not be studied independently of the whole of a drug's action, for this is needed for their interpretation. It is a fact that the study of characteristics alone leads quickly to practical results, but also to permanent mediocrity in knowledge of drug action.

Boeninghausen's method of interpreting symptomatology consists essentially in the selection from the symptoms of the patient, and from those of the drug, of their *elements*, rather than try to obtain the complete symptom, which latter consists of a *seat or location*, a *sensation* and *a modality;* but, in the present incomplete state of our Materia Medica, most of the symptoms are fragmentary, and but few are complete in the above sense. By the use of Boeninghausen's method, these fragmentary symptoms are supplemented by clinical observation of the *curative* effects. A remedy is selected for a case that is found to possess in its symptomatology marked action (1) in a certain *location;* (2) to correspond with *sensation*, and (3) possess the same modality; *without necessarily having in the proving produced the very symptom resulting from the combination.* It is to be inferred that a *full* proving *would* have it, however. For instance, a patient with a bearing pain in the left hip, relieved by motion, greatly worse in the afternoon, would receive Lycopodium, not because Lycopodium has so far produced in the healthy such a symptom, but because, from the study of its symptoms as recorded in the Materia Medica, we do find that it affects the left hip prominently (locality); that its pains, in various parts of the body, are "tearing" (sensation); and that its general symptoms are relieved by motion and aggravated in the afternoon (modality.) The only justification for such analysis and synthesis of symptoms is the imperfection and limitation of our provings and especially the success following the application of the newly constructed symptom, out of these elements, in removing similar symptoms in the patient, hence in curing, and the reasonableness of the presumption that future, complete provings will develop the missing links of the complete symptom of the drug. It is in entire harmony with the fact that every genuine symptom has these three factors—locality, sensation, and modality—these, when combined, constitute a perfect symptom. It is not usual to get these, in any one symptom, from any one prover, but they may be found scattered through the various provings; hence the legitimacy of Boeninghausen's method.

Read in this connection:

T. F. Allen's paper before the World's Medical Congress at Chicago, 1893, entitled, "The Selection of the Homœopathic Remedy, especially in regard to Boeninghausen's Method," published, with discussions, in *North American Journal of Homœopathy*, August, 1893.

For further practical illustration of the use of Boeninghausen's method see an instructive, analytical report of a case of "Progressive Muscular Atrophy Cured with Phosphorus," by T. F. Allen, reported in *Hahnemannian Advocate*, July 15, 1896.

For further study, consult

"Organon," §§ 153, 164, 165, 178.

Also, the preface to Hering's "Guiding Symptoms," Vol. I.

"Hirschel's Rules and Examples for the Study of Pharmacodynamics," Thos. H. Hayle.

CHAPTER VI.

DRUG RELATIONSHIP.

The study of drug pathogenesy, and its application to the treatment of disease, is furthered by the recognition of different relationships that drugs occupy to each other. Among these, the most apparent, but of least practical value, therapeutically, is the

Family relation, or collateral, side relation (congeners), such as belong to the same, or allied botanical family, or chemical group; thus similarity in origin is its claim. In a very broad way, drugs may be divided, according as they belong, to one of the three kingdoms of nature, thus drugs from the animal kingdom, vegetable or mineral. It is not difficult to note certain great features, common to drugs, belonging to one kingdom; but similarity of effects is more marked as different members of a botanical family, or chemical group, are examined. Thus the Ranunculaceæ family, comprising drugs like Aconite, Pulsatilla, Cimicifuga, etc., show certain symptoms of marked similarity—a family likeness not to be mistaken. This is sometimes so great as to seem identical. For instance, in the case of Ignatia and Nux vomica. Both come from the same order of plants, both contain Strychnia, to the presence of which, undoubtedly, this similarity in effect can be attributed. Now, when this similarity approaches identity of effects, it has been found *that they do not follow each other well.* For instance, in a given case of stomach disorder, indicating Nux vomica, it is injudicious practice to follow this by Ignatia, on account of its too close resemblance to the symptoms of the former remedy, the results being unfavorable, disturbing rather the normal evolution of the curative influence.

Antidotal Relation. Certain drugs antidote each other therapeutically, because they produce similar effects locally in certain parts of the organism or on certain tissues and functions or generally throughout their action as a whole. The antidotal relation is based therefore on similarity and is operative according to the law of cure, similia similibus; and again the antidotal relationship between drugs may be general or partial, according as the similarity in their action is general or confined to certain parts only. Thus camphor antidotes the effects of cantharis only so far as these concern the mucous membrane of the urinary tract, while the same tissue elsewhere is not antidoted by it.

Such antidotal relation is of use in practice, by which we can modify or annul an undesirable action of a drug, for instance, Anacardium bears an antidotal relation to Rhus, especially in its action on the skin, Hepar to Mercury, Chamomilla to Coffea and Pulsatilla, etc. An interesting phase of the antidotal relationship is the mutual antidotal or at least modifying power of the higher and the lower attenuations of the same drug, as well as the antidotal relationship between the chronic effects of the crude drug and the attenuated drug, as is seen in treating chronic tobacco poisoning with Tabacum high. This holds true at times in acute conditions as has been frequently verified in poisoning with Rhus where a high attenuation will prove the quickest antidote.

Concordant or Compatible Relationship. Hahnemann first made the valuable, practical observation that certain remedies act better when they are given in a certain series. There seems to be an affinity between them. They are not of the same natural family, but of wholly dissimilar origin; but they have marked similarities in action. Such remedies may follow each other well; they point to a deeper and closer relationship than that of mere family, or similarity in origin. Such relationship exists, for example, between China and Calcarea, Pulsatilla and Sepia, Belladonna and Mercurius, Nitric acid and Thuja, Mercurius and Sulphur, etc.

Complementary Relation exists between drugs that complete a cure that is begun by another and carried to a certain point, where it is taken up by another drug and completed. If a remedy is allowed its full time of action, it will often lead up to a complementary remedy—that is, the symptoms remaining untouched, or brought to the surface, will often suggest a drug known to be complementary to the one given. This useful relationship of certain group of drugs is of great service in the treatment especially of chronic diseases. Such relationship exists between Belladonna and Calcarea; Apis and Natrum muriaticum; Aconitum and Sulphur; Chamomilla and Magnesia phosphorica; Thuja and Silica.

Inimical relation is the very opposite of the concordant and complementary. There seems to be a lack of harmony between certain drugs, as is also seen in certain chemical affinities. This may be so marked that when following each other in the treatment of a case, disturbance shows itself and the cure is interfered with and the whole case mixed up. Such a relation seems to exist between Apis and Rhus, between Causticum and Phosphorus; Mercurius and Silica; Sepia and Lachesis and others. *Do not give these remedies after each other.* It is well to note these inexplicable conditions of drug action, based on friendly or inimical relationship. If it be remembered that drugs are embodied forces, distinct entities with distinct powers to modify human life as manifested in functional activity and organic changes we can readily see that certain forces can work advantageously side by side; their joint result, thus following each other, being greater than either one singly; and again certain others cannot do so, but mere contact or propinquity upsetting the orderly progress of the case.

For further study see Boeninghausen, "The Sides of the Body and Drug Affinities."

Mohr, "The Inimical Relationship of Drugs."

Hering's contributions in the *Archiv*.

"Farrington's Clinical Materia Medica." Lecture I.

CHAPTER VII.

THE APPLICATION OF HOMŒOPATHY.

Homœopathy consists essentially in the application of the principle of similars. *Drug selection* alone constitutes Homœopathy. The homœopathic physician has to deal with two sets of phenomena in treating disease. On the one hand the patient, with a certain train of morbid symptoms; on the other, similar symptoms known to be produced in the healthy by some drug. The closer this correspondence in its essential features, the more certain and speedy the cure, on the principle that two like and similar forces may neutralize each other. This necessitates consideration of—

1. The examination of the patient, and the record of his symptoms.
2. The selection of the remedy corresponding to this totality of symptoms.
3. The administration of the single remedy.
4. The dose and its repetition.

The Examination of the Patient. The first duty of the homœopathic prescriber is clearly to understand the nature of the disturbed functions of the patient, to get at the full facts of the case so far as they are expressed by symptoms. The examination that elicits them must be thorough and complete, and will yield satisfactory results according to the perfection of the physician's general medical knowledge. His knowledge of anatomy will enable him to detect abnormal conditions of organs; physiology will show abnormal performance of function; chemistry, microscopy, etc., will discover morbid secretions and excretions, etc. He makes use of all instruments that modern science places at his disposal, from the clinical thermometer to the stethoscope, and all other instruments of precision of modern diagnostic skill. All the results thereby attained furnish him with the *objective phenomena* which the patient presents. These go far to establish the *diagnosis* of the pathological condition. The totality of symptoms ascertainable, with the help of our numerous diagnostic aids, furnishes a much more complete picture, analytically, than was possible in Hahnemann's time, when the main reliance had to be placed on the subjective symptoms. These latter are still of paramount importance in deciding between drugs that are capable of producing a similar change in the organism; they thus serve to determine the one most nearly indicated remedy from among a group of more or less related remedies.

The totality of the symptoms must be the sole indication to determine the choice of a curative remedy.

Hahnemann's teaching on this point is expressed in § 18 of the Organon, as follows:

"It is then unquestionably true that, besides the totality of symptoms, it is impossible to discover any other manifestation by which diseases could express their need of relief; hence, it undeniably follows that the totality of symptoms observed in each individual case of disease, can be the *only indication* to guide us in the selection of a remedy."

And, again, in § 70, he says: "All that a physician may regard as curable in diseases, consists entirely in the complaints of the patient and the morbid changes of his health perceptible to the senses—that is to say, it consists entirely in the totality of symptoms through which the disease expresses its demand for the appropriate remedy; while, on the other hand, every fictitious or obscure, internal cause and condition, or imaginary, material, morbific matter are not objects of treatment."

The totality of the symptoms consists in the systematic ascertaining of all the symptomatic facts necessary to determine the curative remedy. The totality of symptoms includes every change of state of body and mind that we can discover or have observed, or that has been reported to the physician; thus, every deviation from health. It includes every subjective symptom that the patient can describe correctly and every objective symptom the physician can discover by his senses, aided by all diagnostic instruments. In examining the patient, a definite, *systematic* plan should be followed. The *regional* plan, the Hahnemannian Schema form, is perhaps the best, as it follows a natural, anatomical arrangement.

Special Precautions to be Observed. Be patient in getting at the symptoms, especially in chronic diseases. There is a great difference between patients; some cannot, others will not, give much aid in analyzing their case; some are morbidly desirous of imparting symptoms and will perhaps, unconsciously, warp their statement by exaggeration.

Do not interrupt the patient in his first recital too much; lead him on, if he wanders off. When he has finished, cross-examine him, by careful questioning, to supply any deficiencies.

Avoid asking leading questions, as far as possible, and not so that the patient must answer yes or no.

Accept no diagnostic suggestions, or pathological theories, or former opinions of other physicians, as these can be no guide for the selection of a curative remedy.

Be sure and get the modalities, especially the influence of the times of day, weather, season, position of body, exercise, sleep, etc.

Pay special attention to the mental state of the patient and his intellectual functions.

Take the apparent, immediate cause of his sickness into special account; this is often of importance for selecting the remedy, even long afterwards.

In chronic diseases, especially, investigation should be extended to the family history of the patient; heredity is a potent factor in determining disease.

The history of the patient's previous diseases, particularly eruptions of any kind that may have been treated with strong local remedies and so suppressed; also, as to all forms of local treatment generally, and the patient's medical habits, the use of patent medicines, purgatives, mineral waters, etc.

Notice any alternation of groups of symptoms, such as gastric and rheumatic symptoms, rheumatic and catarrhal, bronchial and skin affections, etc.

Remember that certain bodily conditions have certain mental states—depression and constipation, anxiety and heart affections, hopefulness and consumption, etc.

Remember that, when a certain train of symptoms are present in some one organ or apparatus of the body, there are almost sure to be present certain other symptoms, objective and subjective, in other organs often, anatomically, quite remote, and of which the patient probably is hardly aware until his attention is called to them by the physician.* For instance, certain pains in the head co-exist with certain uterine affections, or anomalies of vision, etc.

Write down the record of the symptoms, beginning a new line with every symptom. This will greatly facilitate study and reference to allied remedies.

Subjective symptoms are a description by the patient of his feelings as they appear to him—his sensations. The ability to express and describe sensations is not common to all patients; and hence, subjective symptoms must always be interpreted by the physician to a large extent. The patient may deceive his physician in stating them, as is frequently the case with hysterical subjects, or he may not be able to describe them accurately enough to be utilized, as in the case of young children.

Objective symptoms are, as a rule, the most important. They are all such as the physician can ascertain by means of his senses, aided and unaided.

In many phases of disease, and with children and frequently in old people, where organic changes can go on to an alarming extent without very marked, subjective disturbance, objective symptoms are all we practically have on which to base a prescription. In mental diseases, objective symptoms are most important for purposes of prescribing.

Objective symptoms are of special value when they occur during sleep, as then the system is relaxed.

Objective symptoms that are *not specially diagnostic* of the disease, or of some pathological state, when present, are important for purposes of prescribing. On the other hand, objective symptoms that are diagnostic of certain pathological, states, so-called *pathognomonic symptoms*, are of great importance in guiding to a certain *class* of remedies and excluding other groups, even though such may seem superficially indicated.

The Totality in Acute Diseases. In the treatment of acute diseases, much of this investigation is necessarily dispensed with, the physician learns to use his eyes and other senses intuitively and thus to get hold of certain characteristic conditions quickly that are known to correspond to certain remedies. Epidemic conditions come to his aid here for rapid and usually successful prescribing.

The Collective Totality of Epidemic Diseases. During the prevalence of epidemic diseases, colds, grippe, eruptive diseases, etc., it is often the case that two or three remedies cover the field. It is needless to go into every detail of the symptomatology, since the epidemic remedies, when found, correspond to the *collective totality* of numerous cases and types of the epidemic disease; each single case of an epidemic disease presenting only a partial picture of the true totality of the epidemic.

Interpretation of the Totality. Having taken a full stock of the case and thereby obtained the totality of symptoms, before prescribing the homœopathically indicated remedy, correct all hygienic, dietetic and sanitary errors. Often a change in the mode of life or abstinence from some hurtful article of diet will be all that is necessary. But after these things have been attended to, whatever symptoms remain will call for medical treatment.

Having obtained a record of the totality of symptoms, a winnowing process must be instituted, by eliminating the *general* symptoms and interpreting the totality according to the relative value of the symptoms, and thus individualize the case under treatment.

In § 83, Hahnemann says: "Individualization in the investigation of a case of disease, demands, on the part of the physician, principally unbiased judgment and sound sense, attentive observation and fidelity in noting down the image of the disease." Hahnemann's first rule here is that the characteristics of the case must be similar to the characteristics of the drug. § 153. The more prominent, uncommon and peculiar features of the case are specially and almost exclusively considered and noted, for *these, in particular, should bear the closest similitude to the symptoms of the desired medicine,* if that is to accomplish the cure. By this individualization, then, we eliminate the general symptoms common to similar pathological conditions, and present to view the individual patient as the pathological process affects *him.* The morbid forces of the disease unite themselves more or less with the inherent weaknesses and disease tendencies, hereditary or acquired, of the individual and give us his peculiar and therefore characteristic symptoms.

Characteristic or Peculiar Symptoms. Hahnemann calls especial attention to the "more striking, singular and uncommon, peculiar signs and symptoms of a case of disease" which are chiefly to be kept in view. These symptoms of themselves may be of no special value, but become valuable or characteristic by their conditions of aggravation or amelioration, their concomitants or locality. Transient odd and peculiar symptoms are however not so important as such as affect the patient's general condition, hence the modalities, conditions of aggravation and amelioration effects of heat, cold, weather, position, times of day, etc , are most important. *The modalities of a drug are the pathognomonic symptoms of the Materia Medica.*

Mental symptoms of drugs are most important, and are a very pronounced feature in the pathogenesis of certain drugs. Notice the mental state of the patient particularly; does he suffer patiently or otherwise. They are also of great importance prognostically; improvement in the mental condition often precedes bodily and general improvement.

First, or Oldest, Symptoms. In the treatment of chronic diseases, the first indications of a departure from health are of the greatest value, particularly those occurring before there was any treatment. After a remedy has been given, and old symptoms reappear in the inverse order of their development, it is an indication that the cure is progressing favorably, and no other medicine should be given. So, also, in acute diseases, the value of first symptoms is great. In diphtheria for instance, the side upon which it begins may decide the choice of the remedy.*

Etiological Factors. As a further aid in arriving at a utilizable totality of symptoms, the immediate cause of the present illness, if determinable, or its exciting factor, will be a great aid in the selection of the remedy. Such causes may be remote in time, and not of any apparent connection with the present state. This Hahnemann also teaches in § 5, Organon, as follows: "The physician, in curing, derives assistance from the knowledge of facts concerning the most *probable cause* of acute disease, as well as from the most significant points in the entire history of a case of chronic disease; aided by such knowledge he is enabled to discover the primary cause of the latter, dependent mostly on a chronic miasm." This gives, on the one hand, an important place to the *first*, or oldest, symptoms and to causes however remote; and, on the other, it elevates to commanding importance, signs of constitutional defects, the underlying psoric conditions. Unquestionably, such frequently modify and relegate to comparative insignificance symptoms of acute disorder, and favor the selection of a deep-acting, anti-psoric remedy even in acute diseases. Such a selection would be justified by its relationship to a truer similarity than would be expressed by an uninterpreted totality of symptoms.

Late Symptoms. The more recent symptoms are valuable as being the latest expression of the diseased

---

condition, and must be covered by the remedy. This is especially true in acute diseases. This is so when another remedy is chosen; the last symptoms that appear must be the guide to it. Again, if a patient has been drugged by palliative medication, we must direct our antidotes principally against the drugs given last —for instance, against Quinine, Pulsatilla, Ipecac, etc.; against Iodine, Hepar; against Chloroform, Hyoscyam, etc. But this rule should not be applied too rigorously; it is best to give no medicine at all for a time.

Functional symptoms of an affected organ are of much less value than symptoms which occur in other parts during the exercise of the function of that organ. Burning pain in the urethra, during or after micturition, is of little value in gonorrhœa, for it is usually present; but pain in the testicles, thighs, or abdomen during or after micturition, or symptoms of some other part not immediately concerned in that function, would be more important. So, also, pain in the stomach after eating, in indigestion, is not of as much value as vertigo or headache after eating would be in the same attack. Therefore, symptoms that affect the general organism are of more value than those that are functionally related to the organ affected.*

Need of Pathology. A knowledge of the pathology of disease (not mere passing, pathological theories, against which Hahnemann so justly protested,) is necessary to interpret the symptomatology obtained and prescribe the truly indicated remedy, and not merely one *externally* homœopathic. The true meaning of any symptom is reached not by considering it alone, but by viewing it in relation to all the rest, and thus placing it in its proper relative position. We must

* S. Kimball.

learn to view symptoms in perspective. The natural history of diseases must be learned, as well as their different stages and characteristic signs accompanying them.

The use of pathology in interpreting the symptoms is seen in the treatment of a case of typhoid fever, where the fever, restlessness, etc., might call to mind Aconite as a remedy; but a little closer examination would show this to be but a partial and apparent homœopathic relationship. Pathology would interpret the fever and restlessness of the typhoid patient and associate them with the coming prostration, the septic condition, the asthenia—conditions wholly foreign to Aconite, which can deal only with sthenic inflammations and healthy blood.

Some symptoms are primary, others reflex. After an organic disease has become established, secondary modifications of health take place, which do not offer valuable symptoms for purposes of prescribing the curative remedy. Really valuable guiding symptoms, if found at all, will be in the *earlier* state of the patient *before* the organic changes have taken place; thus, in the treatment of an organic kidney disease, a curative remedy would be more likely to be found in the earlier symptoms that preceded the development of the dropsy, anemia, etc., characteristic of the later stages.

Pathology also teaches the important difference between the absolute, pathognomonic symptoms and the contingent or peculiar symptoms of a given case of disease.

General or absolute symptoms are those which are common to all patients suffering from the same disease and *they are essential for purposes of diagnosis.* Thus the fever, sore throat and rash are general or absolute symptoms of Scarlatina, while again, the fever, cough, physical signs and bloody sputa are absolute symptoms of Pneumonia.

Contingent or peculiar symptoms are those which vary with the individual and are not essentially pathognomonic of the *disease*, but always of the individual patient. They are therefore the characteristic symptoms of the patient's totality of symptoms, and hence most essential in selecting the remedy. Hence the rule:

The greater the value of a symptom for purposes of diagnosis, the less its value for the selection of the homœopathic remedy and vice versa.

The seemingly unimportant, peculiar, contingent symptoms of the patient, though valueless for purposes of diagnosis, are the chief guiding symptoms for the selection of the homœopathic remedy.

Totality of quality rather than of quantity, is the basis for homœopathic prescribing. In any case of disease it is necessary to discover in what way, that is, by what peculiar symptoms, does one case of illness differ from every other of the same disease. How does *this* patient's typhoid or rheumatism differ from the typhoid or rheumatism of every other patient. This special totality of quality, or of characteristics will unerringly lead to the curative homœopathic remedy. This is the *Hahnemannian Similarity*. It exists between the *characteristic* symptoms of the *patient* and the *characteristic* symptoms of the *drug*, and we must *individualize each case* in order to arrive at this desirable goal, for the selection of the hemœopathic remedy. This differs from the mere *Pathological Similarity* which consists in matching diseased conditions or pathological processes as determined by pathological anatomy. It adapts the remedy to a *disease* rather than to the *individual patient*.

Thus, in the treatment of pneumonia, a remedy would be given that actually produces lesions similar to the pneumonic process. Phosphorus has actually produced hepatization of the lungs in animals poisoned by it; hence, it should be the curative similar, as it is undoubtedly the pathological similar. So Arsenic produces a gastro-enteritis and ultimate lesions just like cholera, and should, therefore, be the curative remedy in this disease, since it is the pathological similar. But experience denies this deduction. To be curative, a remedy must correspond to the characteristic symptoms, whether these are based upon the ultimate pathologico-anatomical lesion or not. Unquestionably, the similarity in pathological process or lesion is one of the most important factors in the totality, but not the determining one in every case.

Examples of pathological similarities between diseases and drugs. The gastro-enteritis and paralysis of Arsenic; epileptiform convulsions of Hydrocyanic acid; broncho-pneumonia of Tartar emetic; anæmia of Argentum; catalepsy of Cannabis indica; tinnitus aurium of Quinine; Meniere's disease of Salycilic soda; colic of Plumbum; asthma of Ipecac; tabes of Ergot; fatty degeneration of Phosphorus; glycosuria of Uranium; meningitis of Belladonna, etc, etc.

Use of Pathological similarity. Often in the course of acute diseases, and in children, where no characteristic symptoms can be obtained, pathological correspondence may be the only recourse; but it is otherwise in the treatment of most chronic diseases. Here the method of the Hahnemannian similarity yields best results.

Method of Treating Slight Ailments. It is a mistake to prescribe remedies for every slight ailment. It is best to follow Hahnemann's directions, Organon, § 150: "Whenever a patient complains of only a few insignificant symptoms of recent origin, the physician is not to regard them as a disease requiring serious medical aid. A slight change of diet and habits of living generally suffices to remove so slight an indisposition.

Absence of Characteristic Symptoms in the Totality. There are cases where it is almost impossible to obtain any very characteristic symptoms; these are difficult to handle. § 165. Or there may be only one or two prominent symptoms, which may obscure the remaining features of the case, so-called

Partial or One-sided Diseases. The best rule is to be most painstaking in eliciting symptoms, and then make the best uses of the few symptoms to serve as guides in the selection of the remedy. Although the remedy may be but imperfectly adapted, it will serve the purpose of bringing to light the symptoms belonging to the disease, thus facilitating a choice of the next remedy. Organon, §§ 173–184. Diagnostic symptoms of a disease, although of least importance for selecting the remedy, may be all we have in a given case for guidance. If so, the remedy corresponding to them can be chosen by paying special attention to their modalities, *i. e.*, conditions of aggravation, concomitants, etc. For instance, in dysentery, the tenesmus is an important, diagnostic symptom, but no guiding one to any remedy, since many medicines have this general symptom; but if attended with any modalities or concomitants, it may become a leading indication; for instance, *Nux vom.*, the tenesmus and pain in the back cease with the stool; in *Mercurius*, they continue after it. In this way a general symptom may become a characteristic one, leading to the choice of the curative drug.

For further study consult:

"Organon," §§ 153–173.

"The Relative Value of Symptoms," by S. A. Kimball, M.D., in *Homœopathic Physician*, June, 1895. A very valuable essay.

"The Examination of the Patient for a Homœopathic Prescription," by P. P. Wells, M.D. Transactions Int. Homœopathic Association, 1888, page 18.

"The Genus Epidermicus," by A. McNeil, M.D. Transactions of Hahnemann Association, 1889.

"The Selection of the Homœopathic Remedy," by T. F. Allen, M.D. Read before World's Medical Congress in Chicago, 1893; published in *North American Journal of Homœopathy*, August, 1893.

"The First Prescription," by O. M. Drake, M.D., in *Homœopathic Physician*, January, 1895.

"Dudgeon's Lectures on Homœopathy." Lecture XI: On the Selection of the Remedy. This gives an account of the different views held by the representative older disciples of Hahnemann, and is very interesting from an historical point of view.

"The Totality of Symptoms." A paper read before the American Institute of Homœopathy, by Wm. Boericke, M.D. Published in the *Hahnemannian Advocate*, August, 1896.

CHAPTER VIII.

THE SIMILIMUM.

The indicated remedy in any case is the remedy that corresponds to the totality of symptoms, as interpreted according to the relative rank of symptoms, and not one covering, merely some isolated characteristic or key-note symptom, or, on the other hand, one that corresponds merely to the pathological lesion. The objections to the key-note system of selecting the remedy are its disregard for the full study of the remedy and elevation, instead of some minor often clinical symptom, yielding at best only palliative results, while the objection to the pathological basis is its incompleteness, being only a partial picture of the totality of symptoms and therefore an unreliable basis for curative prescribing.

The similimum is the most similar remedy corresponding to a case, one covering the true totality of symptoms, and when found, is always curative, and in incurable cases, it is the best possible palliative remedy.

Unfortunately, in the present state of our Materia Medica, and other limitations of our art, the Similimum in any case of illness, is not always discoverable. Nevertheless, a cure is possible, albeit, not so prompt as it would be if the chosen remedy were the Similimum to the case. While this is the ideal to be sought, the prescriber must more frequently be satisfied with the selection of a mere *similar* instead. Fortunately, the very conception of similarity is one of *relative* nearness and does not express an *absolute* relation; it is comparative always, thus a drug is more or less similar according to the nearness of its correspondence to the totality of symptoms. Moreover, the experience and practice of the homœopathic school teaches that any one of several more or less similar remedies may be used with alike good results, that is, it may be sufficiently similar to bring about nature's reaction.

The merely similar remedy, though falling short of the dignity of the Similimum is not thereby removed from capacity of curative service, but the curative response is not as direct and prompt as results from the administration of the similimum which must ever be, in every homœopathic prescription, the ideal to be sought.

The selection of the Similimum involves its administration singly and without admixture of any other medicinal substance.

The single remedy is the necessary corollary to the similar remedy. It is to be given alone, not alternated or mixed with any other*. Only then can its pure effects be evolved and estimated, and the single remedy must be given in the smallest dose that will bring about nature's reaction. The single remedy does not mean a simple remedy. All chemical salts, which are composite substances, the juice of plants, like Opium, a most marvelously compounded substance, are all single remedies and used as such in homœopathy. Any single substance *that has been proved upon the healthy*, as an entity and whose pathogenesis is known, can be administered; but it must be given unmixed with any other medicinal substance, so as to obtain its own peculiar drug force unmodified by any other.

It is the similar relationship alone that constitutes the homœopathicity. The size of the dose has com-

* As early as 1797, Hahnemann wrote, in *Hufeland's Journal*, that for several years he had never administered anything but the *single* remedy at a time, and never repeated the dose until the action of the first had expired.

paratively little to do with it, except so far as experience may indicate it. It may be given in a crude form, wholly unprepared by the pharmacist's skill, or in material dosage, provided it does not produce temporary aggravation of the symptoms; or it may be administered stripped of all its apparent material, visible and tangible particles. Experience alone can teach which will bring about the best results in any given case.

Alternation or rotation of remedies is reprehensible practice, since it leads away from accurate and definite knowledge of drug effects, and sooner or later leads to polypharmacy, which is the most slovenly of all practice. Since we have no provings of combination of drugs, it would be impossible to prescribe such combinations with scientific accuracy. In regard to alternation, Hahnemann says: "Some homœopathists have made the experiment in cases where they deemed one remedy suitable for one portion of symptoms of a case of disease, and a second for another portion, of administering both remedies at once, or almost at once; but I earnestly deprecate such hazardous experiments, that can never be necessary, though they sometimes seem to be of use." Note to § 272, Organon.

For further study, read—

"Organon," §§ 272–275.

Dunham: "Science of Therapeutics—Alternation of Remedies."

Edmund Capper: "The Method of Hahnemann and the Homœopathy of To-day," in *Journal of British Homœopathic Society*, January, 1895.

Jones: "The Ground's of a Homœopath's Faith." Lecture 2: "The Single Remedy."

Joslin: "The Principles of Homœopathy—The Single Remedy."

Eleanor F. Martin, M.D.: "The Single Remedy *vs.* Alternation," in *Pacific Coast Journal of Homœopathy*, October, 1894.

CHAPTER IX.

THE SECOND PRESCRIPTION.

In the treatment of chronic diseases, Hahnemann's instructions to *write out* the symptoms and arrange them according to the rules given, is an absolute necessity to attain accuracy of knowledge of the possible indicated drugs and the selection of the most similar remedy. This procedure ensures also a ready selection of the *second* prescription, since the record will answer all of the necessary questions and determine the right course to be pursued. The prescriber's attitude after the first prescription, in the treatment of chronic diseases especially, ought to be passive. The first and foremost rule is *to wait and watch further developments.* The selected homœopathic remedy simply stimulates the vital forces to reaction, and we must await results.

No further interference is called for when any one of the following conditions presents itself:

1. *Short aggravation of the Symptoms.* This is a curative effect of the remedy. Do not interfere with it unless the aggravation continues and the general state of the patient is worse, in which case an antidote, *i. e.*, a homœopathic remedy for the latest symptoms is indicated. Usually one dose of such an antidote is all that is required to modify the condition, and then the case can progress without further interruption.

2. *General Amelioration of the Symptoms.* It is self evident that such a condition should not be disturbed by further medication, on the principle of letting well enough alone. If the disease gets better from within outward, from above downward from more vital to less vital parts, the improvement is permanent and radical.

So an improved mental state is always a favorable indication of a well chosen remedy.

3. *Reappearance of old Symptoms.* The return of some of the older symptoms, if not too severe, indicates a curative action of the remedy administered, if they *appear in the reverse order of their development, i. e.,* if the latest symptoms disappear first.

4. *Appearance of new symptoms.* If such come on after the administration of a remedy, they may be clinical symptoms of the remedy, and if there is at the same time *general improvement,* they need not be considered, as they will disappear. If they persist, the homœopathic antidote will soon rectify the passing increase of the morbid phenomena. Under all these conditions, no further medication is required. So long as improvement is thus progressing, it is folly to change the remedy, and it is not advisable even to repeat the dose.

Other Favorable Symptoms. In acute disease, it is a favorable symptom if the patient *falls asleep* soon after taking the remedy; also, if he feels *generally better,* though the local symptoms may not show any improvement. The improvement here is probably largely psychical, and will soon be followed by the necessarily slower improvement on the physical plane.

The mental condition and general hehavior of the patient, if more tranquil and natural, are among the most certain and intelligible signs of incipient improvement, especially in acute diseases.

Should this progressive evolution of the symptoms towards health cease,

A further review of the case is required, and a new remedy is to be chosen when—

(1) The mental state shows an embarrassed, helpless state instead of the tranquility of improvement.

(2) When no change of any kind follows the first prescription, after waiting long enough for reaction, which is, however, a variable matter, according to the chronicity of the case and character of the remedy chosen, the shortest period to be allowed in a chronic disease being one week, and preferably a longer time.

(3) *When new and important symptoms and old modalities, especially aggravations that persist*, characterize the case, proving that the remedy was not homœopathic to the case, and acted only as a pathogenetic agent in producing new symptoms. This is the danger of selecting a remedy only remotely similar instead of the similimum. The second remedy will often be found a complementary drug of the first.

Three Precautionary Rules of Hahnemann. The author of Homœopathy, in his work on "The Chronic Diseases," has established three precautionary rules, which he has impressed in the most urgent manner upon the minds of his disciples, and which no homœopathic physician can violate without committing the greatest faults in practice. They are the following:

1. To suppose that the doses which he had recommended for every anti-psoric remedy, and which experience had taught him to be the proper doses, are too small.
2. The improper selection of a drug.
3. The too great haste in administering a new dose.

Precautionary Rule No. 1.—Smallness of dose. The debates relative to the smallness of doses are far from being closed. The more that has been written on that subject for some years past, the more contradiction has been heaped upon contradiction. What is a truly remarkable circumstance in this discussion—a circumstance which is by no means creditable to the opponents of small doses—is the fact that the manner in which Hahnemann gradually arrived at the introduction of the small doses in practice, in consequence of repeated trials, observations, experience, seems either to have been forgotten or entirely ignored.

It is experience, and nothing else, which led the carefully-observing author of that immortal text-book to that minuteness of doses which has now become an object of derision. In the second edition of "Chronic Diseases," after having spoken of homœopathic aggravations, Hahnemann continues thus: "*If the original symptoms of the disease continue with the same intensity in the succceding days as in the beginning, or if this intensity increases, this is a sure sign that, although the remedy may be homœopathic, yet the magnitude of the dose will make the cure impossible.* The remedial agent, by its powerful disproportionate action, not only neutralizes its genuine homœopathic effects, but established, moreover, in the system, a medicinal disease by the side of the natural disturbance, which is even strengthened by the medicine."

That portion of the preceding quotation, which is printed in italics, embodies a great truth which has never been denied, which has been abundantly confirmed by the numerous results of the allopathic treatment of chronic diseases, and is, therefore, well worthy of attentive and serious consideration. Such results are even witnessed in the comparatively easy treatment of syphilis, from the abuse of mercury, which is then secondary syphilis.

Hahnemann continues afterwards: "This pernicious effect of too large a dose may be observed already in the first sixteen, eighteen or twenty days of its action. In such a case it becomes necessary either to give an antidote, or if the antidote should not be known, to administer a very small dose of such antipsoric as corresponds most homœopathically to the symptoms of both the natural and the artificial disease. If one antipsoric should not be sufficient, another, of course, ought to be given, after having been selected with the same care."

How little an excessive dose is capable of displaying its full curative powers may be seen from the following remarks of the author of homœopathy: "The excessive action of the otherwise homœopathic remedial agent having been subdued by the proper antidote or by antipsoric remedies, the same agent may then be exhibited again, but of a much higher potency, and in a more minute dose." But this agent would have no effect, if a first powerful dose of it had not accomplished in the beginning all the good that the agent is capable of doing.

Finally, Hahnemann observes: "Nothing is lost by giving even smaller doses than those which I have indicated. The doses can be scarcely too much reduced, provided the effects of the remedy are not disturbed by improper food. The remedial agent will act even in the smallest quantity, provided it corresponds perfectly to all the symptoms of the disease, and its action is not interfered with improper diet. The advantage of giving the smallest dose is this, that it is an easy matter to neutralize their effects in case the medicine should not have been chosen with the necessary exactitude. This being done, a more suitable antipsoric may be administered."

This advice ought to be carefully considered, especially by the beginners, together with the warning which Hahnemann has expressed in the preface to his work on "Chronic Diseases." "What would they have risked, if they had first followed my indications and then employed small doses? The worst which would have befallen them was, that those doses would have been of no avail. It was impossible that they should do any harm. But instead of exhibiting small doses, they employed, from a want of sense and of their own accord, large doses for homœopathic use, thus exposing the lives of their patients, and arriving at truth by that circuitous route which I had traveled upon before them with trembling hesitation, but the end of which I had just reached with success. Nevertheless, after having done much mischief, and after having squandered the best period of their lives, they were obliged, when they were really desirous of curing a disease, to resort to the only true method which I had demonstrated to them a long while ago. *

Diet and Regimen during Homœopathic Treatment. Hahnemann and the early homœopathists laid great stress on a strict diet; but this is a field that has been greatly neglected in modern times, largely because it was found that the power and efficacy of the well-chosen remedy were able to manifest themselves, notwithstanding great license in diet and hygiene. Nevertheless, a return to Hahnemann's careful restrictions may be advisable in many cases. His teachings, in this regard, are as follows:

"The minuteness of the dose required in homœopathic practice, makes it necessary that every other kind of medicinal influence that might cause a disturbance should be avoided in the diet and regimen of patients, in order that the highly rarified dose may not be counteracted, overpowered, or disturbed by extraneous, medicinal influences. In chronic cases, therefore, it is especially necessary to remove all obstacles of this nature with the greatest care, since they exercise a deleterious effect."

Regimen in Acute Diseases. Here the instinct of the patient usually guides him aright, and his cravings

* Quoted from Von Boenninghausen.

can be judiciously gratified. "The food and drink most commonly craved by patients suffering from acute diseases is generally of a palliative and soothing kind, and not properly of a medicinal nature, but merely adapted to the gratification of a certain longing."

"In acute diseases, the temperature of the room and the quantity of covering should be regulated entirely according to the wishes of the patient, while every kind of mental exertion and emotional disturbance is to be carefully avoided."

For further study, read:

"Organon," §§ 253–263.

"The Second Prescription," by Dr. J. T. Kent, in Proceedings of the Hahnemannian Association, 1888, page 71.

"Practical Hints on the Management of Chronic Cases." by W. P. Wesselhoeft, M.D., in Transactions of Hahnemannian Association, 1889, page 8.

"Procedure in the Treatment of Inactive, Progressive Chronic Diseases," by T. J. Kent, in *Hahnemanniau Advocate*, July, 1896.

CHAPTER X.

HAHNEMANN'S NOSOLOGY.

The classification of diseases adopted by Hahnemann includes two types, acute and chronic. §§ 72–82, Organon.

Acute diseases originate from defective hygiene, errors in diet, physical agents, cold, heat and other atmospheric changes, mental and moral influences.

Again, telluric and meteoric and bacterial influences give rise to acute diseases, attacking a number of individuals, at the same time giving rise to epidemic and contagious diseases. Besides these general causes, there are types of acute disease that are transient activities of the hitherto dormant psoric miasm, rendered so from some cause or other.

It is well to bear this possible cause of certain acute diseases in mind, since corresponding antipsoric remedies may possibly come into requisition for their cure or temporary subsidence.

Chronic diseases are such as are produced by infection from a chronic miasm, and which the vital powers of the organism, aided by hygienic and dietetic and sanitary measures are not able to extinguish. The chronic miasms giving rise to all forms of chronic disease are psora, syphilis and sycosis. Hahnemann does not classify among these chronic diseases such as result from living under unhygienic and unsanitary influences, or trying mental conditions, dietetic errors, excesses of all kinds, etc. These diseases disappear of themselves by mere change of regimen and surroundings and removing the cause, provided, there is not present one of the three chronic miasms that are the real causes of all chronic disease.

Drug Diseases. On the other hand, prolonged drug use in heroic doses does produce a species of chronic disease that is most difficult to cure, and when such have attained a considerable hold, it would seem as if no remedy could be discovered for their radical cure. * Organon, §§ 74 and 75.

"It is a matter of regret that we are still obliged to count among chronic diseases, very common affections which are to be regarded as the result of allopathic treatment, and the continual use of violent, heroic medicines in large and increasing doses. Examples of that kind are: the abuse of Calomel, Corrosive sublimate, Mercurial Ointment, Nitrate of Silver, Iodine and its ointments, Opium, Valerian, Quinine, Digitalis, etc., the use of purgatives persisted in for years, etc." To which might be added the modern abuse of Coal tar products, patent medicines. Such wanton treatment weakens the organism, abnormally deranged and wholly altered. Irritability and sensibility are increased or decreased, hypertrophy and atrophy, softening and indurations in certain organs and organic lesions are produced. Such are some of the results of nature's efforts to protect the organism against complete destruction by aggressive treatment with pernicious drugs.

The Evolution of Hahnemann's Doctrine of Chronic Diseases. After Hahnemann's discovery of the Law of Cure in 1790, he worked incessantly inves-

---

* The treatment of drug diseases by the use of the highest potency of the drug producing them is to be tried in these obstinate chronic affections, it is an entirely consistent homœopathic procedure.

tigating the action of drugs on the healthy, and practiced according to the newly-discovered law and by the light and aid the new Materia Medica was able to give. The success of this practical application of the Law of Cure was striking in the extreme. Especially true was this in the treatment of acute diseases and epidemics. As to chronic diseases, in which allopathic treatment was so often worse than useless, homœopathy rarely failed to improve or ameliorate the conditions in a very short time. But, though the patients were often very much relieved, they were not cured, for their complaints would return more or less by many unfavorable circumstances, such as errors of diet, poor hygienic conditions, unfavorable weather, mental emotions, etc. Their return, under these circumstances, was generally attended with the appearance of new symptoms, often more troublesome and more difficult of removal than before. Even when the treatment of these chronic diseases was conducted strictly according to the doctrines of the homœopathic art, Hahnemann himself owned that "their commencement was cheering, their progress less favorable, their issue hopeless." "And yet," he adds, "the homœopathic doctrine itself is built upon the impregnable pillars of truth and must ever remain so." Whence this inferior success, this absolute want of success in the prolonged treatment of chronic diseases? If homœopathy is based upon a natural law—*nature's law for healing*—and the conditions for carrying out the law are observed, there ought not to be any failure—only success. Why, then, this failure at times in certain patients and even typical acute diseases; why this almost constant failure in chronic disease?

He says that, from the year 1816–17, the solution of this problem occupied him day and night, and at length he succeeded in solving it. Like all of Hahnemann's work, it was the fruit of long and patient observation and study and experiment.

Ten years later, in 1827, he was ready to communicate this new discovery, as he believed this epoch-making theory, to the profession. He summoned to Coethen, where he was then practicing as physician to the reigning prince, two of his most esteemed disciples, Doctors Stapf and Gross, and communicated to them his theory of the origin of chronic diseases and his discovery of a completely new series of medicines for their cure, exhorting them to test the truth of his opinions and discoveries in their own practice. He disclosed this to these two disciples in case his death—for he was then in his seventy-third year—should have occurred before the publication of his book on the subject. This remarkable book, entitled "The Chronic Diseases, Their Peculiar Nature and Homœopathic Treatment," duly appeared the next year, 1828. With the publication of this book, supplementing the Organon, the high-water mark of medical philosophy was reached. A few generations hence this will be generally acknowledged.

Cause of Recurrence of Chronic Diseases.

His researches and reflections, Hahnemann tells us in his work, led him to the conclusion that the cause of the constant recurrence of chronic diseases after their apparent or partial removal by the homœopathic remedy, and their recurrence with new and grave symptoms, was that the symptoms manifesting themselves at any one time were *only a portion* of the deeply-seated fundamental malady, whose great extent was shown by the new symptoms that appeared from time to time. He believed it to be a chronic miasm, which the body could not throw off spontaneously and unaided, not by careful diet or regimen, but that it rather increased in intensity and extent from year to year.

"The most robust constitution, the best regulated life, and the greatest energy of the vital powers, are insufficient to extinguish them." § 78, Organon.

The Skin Phase of Chronic Diseases.

His further research showed that the obstacle to the cure seemed to lie in a previous scabious eruption, which the patient frequently acknowledged having had, and from which he often dated all his sufferings. He believed that chronic diseases occurred on the suppression artificially, or disappearance from any cause of a scabious, itching, eruption from the skin in otherwise healthy persons. Itch, in Hahnemann's time, was a term which covered many other affections besides the one now known as scabies or itch. This itch dyscrasia he called *Psora*, meaning thereby the internal itch disease, with or without any present skin symptoms. It is the source of all varieties of skin diseases, abnormal growths, tumors, deformity, mental diseases, etc. In short, it is the parent of all chronic diseases, with the exception of venereal diseases. It is the oldest, most universal and obstinate of all miasmatic diseases. The leprosy of the Israelites, the epidemic St. Anthony's fire of the middle ages, were but forms of this taint. In these forms the whole malignity seemed to be expended on the skin. Greater cleanliness and generally better modes of living have modified its local manifestations, so that, at the present day, it is more in herpetic and eczematous diseases that we meet with it. The readiness with which these are suppressed, the readiness with which ordinary practice dries up discharges of all kinds, the immense development of local treatment, and the increase of all kinds of specialists, whose tendency is to suppress local manifestations of disease, has driven this psora within to more vital regions, and thus has lead to the great increase of chronic maladies that afflict mankind.

The appearance of skin symptoms, or discharge from a mucous surface, shows that nature is making an effort to localize on the outskirts of the body the morbid process, removed as far as possible from the more vital parts of the organism, where it would be much more mischievous. Therefore, forcing it back into the interior by strong, local treatment must necessarily work detrimentally to a radical and permanent cure.

" Every external treatment of a local symptom whose aim is to extinguish it on the surface of the body without curing the internal miasmatic disease—such, for example, as that of destroying a psoric eruption on the skin by means of ointments, healing up a chancre by the use of caustic, destroying the granulations of sycosis by ligature, excision or the application of a hot iron—is not only useless, but injurious. This pernicious method, in such general use at the present day, is the chief source of the innumerable chronic diseases that oppress the human race. This is the most criminal practice physicians can adopt, and it has, notwithstanding, been very generally practiced till the present time, and taught, *ex cathedra*, as the only one. § 203, Organon.

The Underlying Facts of the Psoric Theory. Without the necessity of accepting the Psoric doctrine as a whole, the homœopathic school has found in it an excellent working hypothesis, and certain facts are undeniable and go far to establish the essential truth of the doctrine. These are the following:

1. In many patients, the even and regular clinical course of diseases is from some course or other within themselves interfered with.

2. Remedies apparently indicated and chosen according to the law of similars, fail to accomplish what, as a rule, they ought.

3. This is especially true of most chronic diseases.

4. It is a further fact that frequently the suppression or disappearance of a skin disease is followed by serious mischief in more vital organs, as respiratory affections (asthma), after eczema capitis, etc., showing a reciprocal relation between the skin and internal organs.

It is the presence of this unseen but nevertheless very active and perturbing factor that accounts for these conditions. Now, this fact of recognition is the mark of genius. The *theory* of its precise nature is of comparatively little importance and may or may not be true. That it is nothing but suppressed itch in the narrow sense is not true. That, however, suppressed skin affections in a wider acceptation than what we now-a-days understand by itch are an indubitable factor in the production of many forms of obstinate and occult chronic suffering far removed from local skin manifestation, is an established truth. The Hahnemannian conception of Psora is a very real thing, the Psora theory an intensely practical thing and THAT is its passport to the general practitioner whose aim is to cure permanently rather than palliate and relieve for the time being. Perhaps it would have been better not to try and define the inner essence of this dyscrasia. The celebrated Botanist Schleiden, used to open his lectures on Botany by frankly confessing that he did not know what a plant was. So we may not know what Psora is, except that it consists of the sum of all the biological obstacles which resist, deface, complicate and alter the natural course of diseases and interfere with the action of the apparently well selected homœopathic remedy. In this wider sense, as indicating cachexia or dyscrasia, the Psora theory is founded in nature and truth. Though Hahnemann's theory is not proven, it is a most admirable working theory, a stepping stone by means of which we attain remarkable results in the treatment of disease.

Anti-psoric remedies are such as show in their pathogenesis a tendency to act from within outwards, from above downwards, who thus abound in skin symptoms and are deep and long-acting remedies; hence, they are of special value in the treatment of chronic disease and for the eradication of inherited and constitutional disease tendencies. They show their greatest medicinal power in highly attenuated form and do not bear frequent repetition. Many of them are wholly inert in their crude state and require the pharmaceutical processes of homœopathy to develop their latent medicinal force.

The principal anti-psoric remedies are Sulphur, Calcarea, Lycopodium, Sepia, Silica, Natrum mur., Graphites, Arsenic, Alumina, etc.*

Hahnemann's Suggestion in Regard to Administering Anti-psoric remedies. "The best time for

* The following is Hahnemann's list of anti-psoric remedies, but there are quite a number of others that ought to be included, which have been proved and introduced since his time:

Agaricus,	Colocynthis,	Natrum carb.,
Alumina,	Cuprum,	Natrum mur.,
Ammon. carb.,	Digitalis,	Nitric acid,
Ammon. mur.,	Dulcamara,	Petroleum,
Anacardium,	Euphorbium,	Phosphorus,
Antimon. crud.,	Graphites,	Phosphoric acid,
Arsenic,	Guaiacum,	Platina,
Aurum,	Iodum,	Sarsaparilla,
Baryta carb.,	Kali carb.,	Sepia,
Borax,	Kali nitricum,	Silica,
Calcarea carb.,	Lycopodium,	Stannum,
Carbo animalis,	Magnesia carb.,	Sulphur,
Carbo vegetabilis,	Manganum,	Sulphuric acid,
Causticum,	Mezereum,	Zincum.
Clematis,	Muriatic acid,	

taking a dose of an anti-psoric medicine is early in the morning while fasting; no food or drink should be taken within half an hour after. After taking the medicine, the patient should keep perfectly quiet at least a full hour, but without going to sleep, avoiding mental exertion of any kind as well.

"To females, anti-psoric remedies should not be given immediately before or during menstruation, not until four days after the flow has commenced."

Pregnancy offers a most favorable time for the administration of anti-psoric remedies, the organism being then in a specially receptive state for the eradication of chronic and inherited disease tendencies.

During treatment of a chronic disease, do not interfere too readily with the acute sufferings that may arise during the treatment. Often such acute symptoms are really a part of the curative action and hence it would be unwise to interfere with their development.

Other Miasms Recognized by Hahnemann.

In the Hahnemannian pathology of chronic diseases, besides psora, two other miasms, *i. e.* syphilis and sycosis figure as etiological factors. The importance and extent of syphilis as a cause of a distinct miasm does not differ as conceived by Hahnemann from that accepted by modern pathology, but sycosis assumes a distinctive importance peculiar to homœopathy.

Sycosis is the suppression of the gonorrhœal poison in the system. Its main local manifestation is the production of figwarts around the genital region, but its later constitutional symptoms are not confined to any part of the organism but are a general deviation of health.

Hahnemann distinguishes two kinds of gonorrhœa—one comparatively innocent—a urethral, catarrhal inflammation, and the other the sycotic form. In regard to the more common and comparatively innocent form, he says in his "Chronic Diseases": "The miasm of the other common gonorrhœas seems not to penetrate the whole organism, but only to locally stimulate the urinary organs. They yield either to a dose of one drop of fresh parsley-juice, when this is indicated by a frequent urgency to urinate, or a small dose of Cannabis or Cantharis, or of Copaiva, according to their different constitution and the other ailments attending it. These should, however, be always used in the higher and highest dynamizations, unless a psora, slumbering in the body of the patient, has been developed by means of a strongly-affecting, irritating or weakening, old-school treatment. In such a case, frequently, secondary gonorrhœas remain, which can only be cured by anti-psoric treatment."

The sycotic form of gonorrhœa differs in being a much more serious matter. Hahnemann describes it as follows: "The discharge is from the beginning thickish, like pus; micturition is less difficult, but the body of the penis swollen somewhat hard; the penis is also, in some cases, covered on the back with glandular tubercles, and very painful to the touch."

The characteristic features of sycosis are the wart-like, cauliflower excresences around the genitals, soft, spongy, bleeding easily, recurring when violently removed, frequently emitting a specific, fetid fluid.

All heroic, external treatment is forbidden, tending to produce the sycotic diathesis; only the external use of Thuja is permitted. For internal treatment, Thuja is the great anti-sycotic.

The violent suppression of a sycotic, urethral discharge is often followed by chronic suffering, which is characterized by peculiar symptoms and conditions, among which the following have frequently been observed:

Symptoms of Suppressed Sycosis. Great muscular debility is the most characteristic physical sign; anxiety; anguish; fear of associating with strangers; going into a crowd; great irritability; dysmenorrhœa, before, during and after flow, with great debility; *sterility*; inflammation of the Fallopian tubes, ovaries; neurasthenia; asthma; bronchial affections; distorted finger nails, eruption in the palms of the hands; dryness of the hair, etc.; rheumatism setting in shortly after the suppression of the discharge or removal of the warts; ankle and knee are specially affected; pains worse before a storm and during the day.

Eradicative Possibilities of Anti-psoric Treatment. The greatest evil of these miasms, is that they are made organic and rendered permanent by heredity. It is this fact of heredity and the pollution of the vital fluids * entailed thereby that modifies not only the course of acute diseases, but establishes and makes a permanent field for chronic diseases. This hereditary gift and this organized field give rise to certain bodily constitutions and certain dyscrasic conditions. Acute diseases and possibly the action of remedies *run their course in the track marked out by these bodily constitutions*, which again are largely modified by the latent psoric taint.

Every practitioner of experience arrives sooner or later at this fact—namely, that in order to get a true and practical understanding of diseases, the *ground*, the human organization modified more or less by heredity, upon which ground diseases feed, and which is the battlefield of the malignant forces of disease from

---

* "The vaccinated syphilis of one organism passing into another, may not manifest itself by eruption, or chancre or visible syphilitic taint at all, but may fall upon the nervous life and be a raging and unappeasable lust in after life."—J. J. Garth Wilkinson.

without *combining with the impurities within*, the character of this ground must be studied; for, according to its composition, it will certainly modify one way or another the course of diseases that from time to time invade it. The presence of this modifying something—this perturbing and yet determining factor—this *psoric taint*, was recognized by Hahnemann. His facts are true; his theory, true or not, is, nevertheless, an admirable working theory, leading to remarkable, successful results.

Pre-natal Treatment by Means of Anti-psoric Remedies. This is a peculiar field for Homœopathy. By means of the deeply-acting anti-psoric remedies, the lower strata of perverted life where it first establishes itself in impurities in the finest fibres and cellular structures, can be restored. Medicines chosen wisely and given to the expectant mother, can benefit the coming child. Frequently, with the indicated remedy, anatomical and structural deficiencies—as cleft palate, hare lip, eczema, etc.—can be prevented in families where such have appeared, because the taint that gave rise to them in former pregnancies has been neutralized by the timely administration of the homœopathic anti-psoric remedies.

Suggestions for the Treatment of Chronic Diseases.

1. Before beginning the treatment of a chronic disease, it is necessary to inquire carefully if the patient has been infected by venereal disease, and, if so, to institute treatment against such infection; but more frequently it will be found that psora complicates the case.

2. Ascertain, also, the nature of medical treatment that the patient had received, either from drugs or mineral baths, etc., in order to understand the deviations which this treatment had produced in the original disease.

3. Patient's age, mode of living, diet, occupation, domestic circumstances, and even his social position, should be considered, in order to see how the cure may be favored or impeded thereby.

4. Patient's mental condition and temperament should not be overlooked, as it may be necessary to direct or modify his mental state by psychical means.

5. Several interviews may be necessary before the physician will find himself enabled to determine the state of the patient's case as perfectly as possible, and to mark the most conspicuous, characteristic or peculiar symptoms, which alone will guide him to the first anti-psoric, anti-syphilitic or anti-sycotic remedy for the beginning of the cure. §§ 206–209, Organon. *

Partial Diseases and Local Affections. Diseases presenting an insufficient number of symptoms, usually only one or two prominent ones, though comparatively rare, are met with. Here, the first selected remedy will only be partially adopted and will, therefore, excite accessory symptoms, which, however, are not wholly due to the remedy given, but were latent, and the remedy served to arouse them; therefore, the new totality of symptoms will enable the prescriber to discover the truly indicated remedy. Organon, §§ 172–184.

The so-called local affections occupy a prominent place among partial diseases. The term is applied to diseased conditions appearing upon external parts, and are mostly of recent origin and caused by external injury. Affections of external parts, requiring mechanical skill, properly belong to surgery alone; as, for instance, when external impediments are to be removed that prevent the vital force from accomplishing

---

* See, also, Hahnemann's Golden Rule, page 93, and "Chronic Diseases," page 125.

the cure, as the opening of cavities, either for the removal of cumbersome substances, or to form an outlet to effusions, etc. §§ 185–6, Organon.

Besides the local affections, requiring surgical and mechanical treatment, there are *local affections that proceed from an internal morbid state.* Such involve the entire state of health of the whole organism, since all its parts are so intimately connected as to form an indivisible whole in feelings and functions; hence, all curative measures should be planned, with reference to the state of the whole system and by means of internal remedies. This is done most effectually by including the record of the exact state of the local disease to every other change that is perceptible in the state of the patient. All these symptoms ought to be united in one perfect image and a remedy chosen according to this true totality. Organon, §§ 190–193.

Objections to Local Application of a Medicine Simultaneously with its Internal Use. It may seem as if such a practice were conducive to more rapid improvement, but it is objectionable in local affections dependent on some chronic miasm, on account of the more rapid disappearance of the local phase than of the internal disease. This often leads to the deceptive impression that a perfect cure has been accomplished.

The local application of non-homœopathic remedies renders the case even more difficult. Local symptoms should not be obliterated by caustics, escharotics, or by excision, since thereby the symptoms necessary for a choice of a curative remedy are obscured, and, also, the chief evidences of a permanent cure are taken away; for, if the local symptoms disappear after the administration of the homœopathic remedy, we have established evidence of the achievement of a radical cure and of complete recovery from the general disease. §§ 196–200, Organon.

The Local Disease is Nature's Effort to Relieve by Derivation. "When the system is affected with some chronic disease which threatens to destroy vital organs and life itself, and which does not yield to the spontaneous efforts of the vital force, this endeavors to quiet the inner disease, and to avert the danger by substituting and maintaining a local disease on some external part of the body, whither the internal disease is transferred by derivation. In this way, the local affection for a time arrests the internal evil, without, however, being able to cure it, or to lessen it essentially. The fontanels of the old school have a similar effect, in the form of artificial ulcers upon external parts; they soothe internal chronic complaints, but without curing them."

Nevertheless, the local malady is never anything more than a part of the general disease, but it is a part which has become excessively developed in one direction by the vital force, and transported to the surface of the body where there is less danger, in order to lessen the internal morbid process. § 201, Organon.

The mental state and temperament of the patient are often of most decisive importance in the homœopathic selection of a remedy, and should never escape the accurate observation of the physician, as the state of mind is always modified in so-called physical diseases.

Mental Diseases and their Treatment. Most of them are in reality bodily diseases. Certain mental and emotional symptoms are peculiar to every bodily disease; these symptoms develop more or less rapidly, and become predominant over all other symptoms, and are finally transferred, like a local disease, into the invisibly fine organs of the mind, where, by their presence, they seem to obscure the bodily symptoms.

In regard to the totality of symptoms of a case of this kind, *all physical symptoms which prevailed before* the disease assumed the mental form are very essential. Comparison between these early symptoms and their present indistinct remnants, which may occasionally appear during lucid intervals or during transient amelioration of the mental disease, will show the continuance of the physical disease, although obscured. Study §§ 214–220, Organon.

Acute insanity, even though due to latent psora, should not be treated with anti-psoric remedies at once, but met with remedies like Aconite, Belladonna, etc., in highly attenuated doses. After such treatment, anti-psoric remedies, with well regulated diet and habits, will do the rest. In the treatment of insanity, the medicines may be given mixed with the patient's usual drink, without his knowledge, thus obviating every kind of compulsion. Study §§ 221–231, Organon, in this connection.

Intermittent and alternating diseases are such as return at certain periods, or where certain morbid conditions alternate with each other. Such are mostly a product of developed psora.

The symptoms which mark the condition of the patient during the period of intermission should chiefly be taken as guides in selecting the most striking homœopathic remedy.

In intermittents, besides the importance of the apyrexia as offering most guiding symptoms for the selection of the remedy, the stage which is most prominent and peculiar should next be considered. The best time to administer the remedy is a short time after the termination of the paroxysm, when the patient has partially recovered from it. The vital force is then in the most favorable condition to be modified by medicine and restored to healthy action. Anti-psoric remedies will generally be required after other remedies corresponding to the special type of fever have failed to bring about a perfect cure. Study §§ 231–244, Organon.

For further study, consult—

"Hahnemann's Chronic Diseases," translated by Prof. L. Tafel.

"Hahnemann's Chronic Diseases," by C. L. Swift, M.D., in *Homœopathic Physician*, February, 1885.

"Sycosis," by F. S. Keith, M.D., in *Homœopathic Physician*, May, 1895.

"Procedure in the Treatment of Inactive, Progressive Chronic Diseases," by T. J. Kent, in *Hahnemannian Advocate*, July, 1896.

C. W. Wolf: "Homœopatische Erfahrungen. Die Grundvergiftung der Mensch heit." Berlin, F. A. Herbig, 1860.

Dudgeon: "Lectures on Homœopathy." Lectures IX and X. "The Doctrine of Chronic Diseases." These give an historical account of the development of the doctrine and the views of the older homœopathists in regard to it.

CHAPTER XI.

POSOLOGY.

By posology (*posos*-how much) is meant the science of dosage. By *doses* are meant the quantities of drugs that are required to produce effects on the body whether the body is in a state of disease or normal health. In order to produce the *direct* effects of drugs, a definite quantity within a certain range is requisite. This can only be determined by experiment and experience, and differs according to the age, temperament and state of health of the subject. It is known as the *physiological dose*. This use of drugs by means of a definite physiological dosage has nothing to do with their homœopathic use.

Different Effects Between Large and Small Doses. Homœopathy discovered the fact that there is an opposition in effects between very large and small doses. A teaspoonful of wine of Ipecac, causes sickness and vomiting, while drop doses cure the same. Large doses of Opium bind up the bowels, while a small dose has the opposite effect. Large doses of Bryonia act as a drastic, while small have a tendency to promote a torpid state of the intestines. This physiological antagonism between large and small doses of drugs is one explanation made use of in regard to the homœopathic law.

Reasons for the difference in Dosage between Drugs chosen Homœopathically and Antipathically. The reason is found in the fact of the *bodily resistance* which must be overcome by the drug before it can manifest its action. Every living organism is in the constant effort to keep itself intact—automatically and unconsciously to the individual. This protecting sphere of its distinctive life offers resistance to any foreign intruder, which *bodily resistance* to everything that tends to disturb its health must be overcome first of all before the drug can manifest its peculiar power.

The physiological dose of any drug, therefore, must be large enough (1) to overcome the normal body resistance; (2) sufficiently more to produce symptoms.

Reasons Why the Homœopathic Dose is Necessarily Smaller. Because here no bodily resistance has to be encountered, since a similar action is already existing in certain organs and tissues, the *disease* having overcome the resistance offered by the protective sphere of the body, and thus the affected region is exposed to attacks from without. The homœopathic remedy acts upon the very tracts involved, and since the protecting gates are down, a much smaller dose is required. Another reason is the fact that the affected parts are probably rendered hypersensitive by the disease process. This is seen daily in every direction. Take a healthy eye, and it receives the rays of light and responds thereto; but let the same eye be inflamed, and see how exquisitely sensitive it becomes to otherwise natural stimuli. A third reason is that the homœopathic remedy is given singly, without admixture with other drugs; and hence, its action is not interfered with.

Aggravation follows sometimes even a Minute Homœopathic Dose. If so, it indicates that either the dose selected is still too strong, and in that case other symptoms will probably appear, or the remedy chosen was *perfectly* homœopathic to the case and the aggravation would be but very temporary and would be in itself the best possible indication *to do nothing further but wait.*

Should aggravation follow a certain dose, it is a good rule to go higher in the scale of potency.

Historical Development of the Homœopathic Dose. At first, Hahnemann prescribed the usual doses (Ipecac, five grains, Nux four grains, Cinchona Bark one to two drams), he soon found that aggravation would follow such dosage, if they were chosen according to the similar relationship to the diseased process. This led him naturally enough to a reduction of dosage, and as he obtained equally good or better results, he kept on decreasing the amount. Yet the transition from the crude dosage to comparative infinitesimal quantities was quite sudden, within one year from 1798 to 1799, he advocated both. For a quarter of a century, Hahnemann gave his remedies in varying potencies, seldom as high as the thirtieth potency,* more frequently between the first and twelfth potency, sometimes descending to more material quantities.

But after he had incorporated the psora theory into his doctrinal edifice, he fixed upon the thirtieth potency as the uniform standard for the dose of all remedies. This was to be given in globules saturated and subsequently dried. He desired uniformity among homœopathists, "and when they describe a cure, we can repeat it, as they and we operate with the same tools. Thus our enemies will not be able to reproach us with having no fixed normal standard." And at the same time, he disapproved of attenuations beyond the thirtieth in these words: "There must be some end to the thing, it cannot go on to infinity."

Whatever the size of a dose of a homœopathic remedy, there is one point which must characterize it, *i. e.*, it must be *sub-physiological*, that is, just short of *producing* symptoms.

Hahnemann's recommendation of the thirtieth potency as the dose for all remedies and cases has not been followed by the school, and rightly so, because it is wholly arbitary and unphilosophical to adopt one potency for all drugs. The physician must here, as in the selection of the remedy, learn to individualize.

Repetition of Doses. Hahnemann's latest teachings were to give but one dose, and await its full action. There is much to be said in favor of this advice in the treatment of chronic diseases. No doubt young physicians repeat their remedy too often and change too frequently. Too frequent repetition of doses frets the system and hinders the cure. The safest general rules, based upon firm adherence to the law and practiced by the closest prescribers are the following:

1. Give one remedy at a time—the one most clearly indicated by the totality of symptoms.

2. Give it preferably at first in a medium potency with a tendency to go higher.

3. So long as improvement shows itself, do not change the remedy, and better also, do not repeat the dose. Learn to wait, for so long as the disease does not progress any further, after giving the medicine, there is no danger in waiting, not until new indications appear.

4. In acute diseases, the doses may have to be repeated frequently, according to the intensity and severity of the case; as a rule every hour or two is often enough, and in most acute, as often as every five to ten minutes may be necessary, but all medication should cease with commencing improvement.

The following golden rule is given by Hahnemann in his Chronic Diseases, page 156:

"The whole cure fails if the anti-psoric remedies, which have been prescribed for the patient, are not permitted to act uninterruptedly to the end. Even if the second anti-psoric should have been selected with the greatest care, it cannot replace the loss which the rash haste of the physician has inflicted on the patient. The benign action of the former remedy which was about manifesting its most beautiful and most surprising results, is probably lost to the patient forever."

In Organon, §§ 247–8, Hahnemann says: "These periods are always to be determined by the more or less acute course of the disease and by the nature of the remedy employed. The dose of the same medicine is to be repeated several times, if necessary, but only until recovery ensues, or *until the remedy ceases to produce improvement.*" Consult, also, §§ 249–252.

Also, in note to § 246, Hahnemann emphatically teaches that the homœopathic physician is to administer but one most minute dose at a time, and to allow this dose to act and to terminate its action. And he holds that the best dose is the smallest in one of the high potencies (the thirtieth) for chronic as well as acute diseases. But, in many forms of disease, a single dose is insufficient; and "hence, it may undoubtedly be found necessary to administer several doses of the same medicine, for the purpose of altering, pathogenetically, the vital force to such an extent, and to raise its curative reaction to such a degree, as to enable it to extinguish completely an entire portion of the original disease."

In § 245, Hahnemann gives this general rule: "Perceptible and continued progress of improvement, in an acute or chronic disease, is a condition which, as long as it lasts, invariably counter-indicates the repetition of any medicine whatever, because the beneficial effect which the medicine continues to exert is rapidly approaching its perfection. Under these circumstances, every new dose of any medicine would disturb the process of recovery."*

The period between the early dosage of Hahnemann and this final designation of the thirtieth potency, as the standard covered about twenty-five years. He now entered upon an entirely new conception of drugs, as embodied medicinal forces, which could be practically separated from their material particles and imparted by means of his peculiar pharmaceutical procedures to inert substances—hence, the development of

The Theory of Dynamization. The process of succussion and trituration is now said to result, not only in a thorough mechanical admixture, but in "a real spiritualization of the dynamic property—a true, astonishing unveiling and vivifying of the medicinal spirit." And Hahnemann looked upon this process as "among the greatest discoveries of the age."

Hahnemann distinguishes carefully between dilutions, or attenuations, and homœopathic dynamizations. While the former are solutions, retaining less and less of the distinctive physical properties, in the proportion

* "In dealing with so complex an organism as the human body, it is not to be wondered at that such definite rules have not been found invariably to hold good. When we consider the manifold varieties of constitution, the different degrees of excitability, and the peculiar idiosyncrasies that are met with, it would appear highly improbable that any absolute law of universal application would be found to meet all contingencies. This is borne out by the evidence furnished by the fact that the greatest diversity of opinion nowadays prevails as to the question of the dose and its repetition. . . . The question remains, to a great extent, unsettled, and the ideas of many, with regard to it, differ considerably from those of the earlier homœopathists. Observation and experience, however, will, without doubt, lead ultimately to more definite lines of guidance."—EDMUND CAPPER, M. D., *Journal of British Homœopathic Society*, January, 1895.

that they are mixed with the diluting vehicle, the latter he deems real potentiation of the medicinal force inherent in drugs. This he clearly teaches in the preface to the fifth volume of his "Chronic Diseases," as follows: "Homœopathic dynamizations are processes by which the medicinal properties, which are latent in natural substances while in their crude state, become aroused, and then become enabled to act in an almost spiritual manner on our life—*i. e.*, on our sensible and irritable fibre. This development of the properties of crude, natural substances (dynamization) takes place, as I have before taught, in the case of dry substances, by means of trituration in a mortar; but, in the case of fluid substances, by means of shaking or succession, which is also a trituration. These preparations cannot be simply designated as solutions, although every preparation of this kind, in order that it may be raised to a higher potency—*i. e.*, in order that the medicinal properties still latent within it may be yet farther awakened and developed, must first undergo a further attenuation, in order that the trituration or succussion may enter still further into the very essence of the medicinal substance, and may thus also liberate and expose the more subtle part of the medicinal powers that lie hidden more deeply, which could not be effected by any amount of trituration and succussion of the substances in their concentrated form."

Nevertheless, Hahnemann recognized the improbability of any separation of matter and force; hence, in a note to § 280, he calls attention to the truth "that a substance divided into ever so many parts must still contain in its smallest conceivable parts always *some* of this substance, and that the smallest conceivable part does not cease to be *some* of this substance and cannot possibly become nothing."

Possibly the radiant state of matter, as described by

Faraday and Crookes, may give point to an explanation of the process of dynamization, and of the value of succussion, even without dilution, as mentioned by Hahnemann in the following extract note to § 270: "I dissolved a grain of soda in half an ounce of wàter, mixed with alcohol in a vial, which was thereby filled two-thirds full, and shook this solution continuously for half an hour, and this fluid was in potency and energy equal to the thirtieth development of power."

If this be really so, the development of power must be due to succussion, some of the particles having been put into their radiant state of energy.

Hahnemann went further in some directions than any of his followers. His practice of olfaction is probably without any followers at present. In § 288 of the Organon, he mentions it as follows:

"It is especially in the form of vapor, by olfaction and inhalation of the medicinal aura that is always emanating from a globule impregnated with a medicinal fluid in a high development of power, and placed dry in a small vial, that the homœopathic remedies act most surely and most powerfully."

While this may be true theoretically, the practice of the school has not availed itself of it to any extent and it is but fair to know that the suggestion for this practice sprung from a desire to evade the unjust laws prohibiting physicians to dispense their own medicines, for Hahnemann suggests in a letter to one of his disciples in regard to this subject: "The physician would give neither powders himself or prescribe them from the drug shops." *

Hahnemann's Reasons why the Sceptic Ridicules these Homœopathic Attenuations. *First*, because he is ignorant that by means of such triturations, the internal medicinal power is wonderfully developed and is as it were liberated from its material bonds, so as to enable it to operate more penetratingly and more freely upon the human organism. *Secondly*, because his purely arithmetical mind believes that it sees here only an instance of enormous subdivision, *a mere material division and diminution*, wherein every part must be less than the whole, as every child knows; but he does not observe, that in these spiritualizations of the internal medicinal power, the material receptacle of these natural forces, the palpable ponderable matter, is not to be taken into consideration at all; *thirdly*, because the sceptic has no experience relative to the action of preparations of such exalted medical power. (Hahnemann in Lesser Writings, p. 734.)

For further study consult—

"A Complete Historical Review of Hahnemann's Posology," by T. L. Bradford, M.D., in his "Life of Hahnemann," Chapters LXXXII–V.

Dudgeon's Lectures, Chapters XII–XVI, on Dynamization and Homœopathic Posology, in which the opinions of the older representative Homœopathists are given.

J. M. Selfridge, M.D.: "Infinitesimals from a Scientific Standpoint," in *Homœopathic Physician*, February, 1896.

Also, the chapter on Hahnemann's Philosophy, page 109.

CHAPTER XII.

THE PREPARATION OF HOMŒOPATHIC MEDICINES.

Pharmacy is the art of preparing drugs for use, and dispensing them as medicines. The method of preparing medicines for homœopathic use differs in many essential details from that of the old school.

Pharmacopœia. This is an authoritative list of drugs and their preparations recognized and used by the profession, and which have thus become officinal. At present we have in homœopathy three pharmacopœias: the British, the German and the American, not differering greatly. The American Institute of Homœopathy has a committee at work on a new and authoritative work, which will be published shortly, and will unquestionably be the future authority in the homœopathic school.

Medicines. The medicines used in homœopathic practice, and included in its pharmacopœia, are taken from all the kingdoms of nature, and include most of the drugs used by the old school and many others not recognized and known there as possessing any medicinal virtues. The pharmaceutical processes of homœopathy are characterized by a marvelous simplicity and perfection requiring the greatest nicety and care, so that the designation homœopathic has actually come to mean a special degree of fineness of quality.

Essential Conditions for Preparing Homœopathic Medicines. *Accuracy* is the basis of every procedure. Make up your mind beforehand to do everything right or not at all.

Cleanliness. Be exquisitely clean and have vials corks and everything necessary of the finest quality Under no condition use the same vial or cork for two different preparations, or potencies, even of the sam drug. No amount of cleansing will make them fit fo different homœopathic preparations. Absolute cleanliness of utensils and instruments and person is essential

Conscientious care in selecting, handling and storin drugs. Keep them from contact with each other; protect them from vapors, odors, dust; store them in cool dry, airy, darkened, pure place.

Drugs for homœopathic use are taken from th three kingdoms of nature; they are either in a liquid state or dry, soluble or insoluble. In order to conver these drugs into homœopathic medicines, which shal contain all the medicinal powers inherent in the crud substances, and in such a state as will secure thei ready and complete assimilation by the organism, *thre different processes* are made use of, trituration, solution and attenuation, and three vehicles or menstrua ar employed for that purpose—sugar of milk, water, and alcohol.

The Menstrua Used in Homœopathic Pharmacy.

Sugar of milk (Saccharum lactis or Lactose). A product of animal life, one of the constituents of milk obtained by evaporating the whey of the milk. It i of pure white color, faintly sweet taste, should be odorless and non-hygroscopic. For homœopathic use, ough to be re-crystallized, as the ordinary product of th shops is not always perfectly pure. It must be kept in a dry place, as it becomes musty when exposed to dampness. The marvelous sagacity of Hahnemann is seen in his selection of sugar of milk for the process o triturating mineral drugs. No other known substanc could equal the sharp, flinty crystals, in grinding to an inconceivably fine powder hard mineral substances, so that they can be rendered absorbable by the body. Its preservative properties are very great, keeping the minutest particles of triturated metals untarnished by oxidation indefinitely. It is easily made into tablets, which, in their pores, can be made to absorb medicinal, alcoholic solutions.

Alcohol is the most important menstruum used in homœopathic pharmacy; it is seldom pure unless redistilled. Alcohol is formed whenever sugar comes in contact with a fermentable matter in water at a suitable temperature. It may be made from a great number of vegetable substances, that from rye or wheat being the best. Pure Alcohol is a colorless fluid which must not lather when rubbed in the hands and have no disagreeable odor. Strong Alcohol contains about 94 per cent by volume of Ethyl Alcohol. It is used principally in the preparation of tinctures or certain solutions.

Officinal or Dispensing Alcohol is used for making the attenuations and is best adapted for medicating pellets. It contains 88 per cent by volume of Ethyl Alcohol.

Alcohol should be kept in well stoppered bottles and in a cool place.

Distilled Water (Aqua distillata). Common water is always impure for medicinal preparations, being charged with gases, earthly matters, etc. Hence distilled water is essential. The still used should be used for no other purpose whatever. The crucial test of the purity of distilled water is its ability to keep. If it has any kind of odor, or becomes turbid it is unfit for homœopathic preparations. It should be kept in glass-stoppered bottles and only in small quantities as it is very liable to deterioration from the entrance of inorganic dust and microbes.

Distilled Water is used as a solvent for many chemical substances; for making solutions of acids, and also converting triturations into liquid attenuations, as is done with all minerals, chemical salts and all other drugs first prepared by triturating them, after the third centesimal poteney.

The Unit of Medicinal Strength. The *dry, crude drug, is the unit of medicinal strength, or drug power.* It is the starting point from whence to calculate the strength of every preparation, be it tincture, solution or trituration. In making triturations or solutions of chemical substances, the matter is very simple, the first potency being the $\frac{1}{10}$ or $\frac{1}{100}$ of the crude drug according to the decimal or centesimal scale. In the case of tinctures, the dry drug also is the unit of drug power, but as this is soluble in varying proportions in different plants, the drug-power of the tinctures varies accordingly.

Preparations of Drugs.

General rule. All substances soluble in either Alcohol or water, are properly made into solutions or tinctures; all insoluble or only partially soluble substances should first be made into triturations only.

Aqueous Solutions are made from such chemicals as are soluble in water. Hygroscopic substances, such as some of the potash and soda preparations ought to be so prepared in the lower potencies in preference to triturating them. The solutions are made in the proportion of one in ten, one in one hundred and one in one thousand, depending upon the degree of the solubility of the substance. Such solutions are as a rule unstable and do not keep for any length of time, and ought, therefore, be renewed whenever required. The solution must be clear, free from sediment and cloudiness.

Tinctures. Homœopathic tinctures are made from plants and other substances wholly or partially soluble in Alcohol. They are, therefore, alcoholic solutions of solids or semi-solids. The chief source of homœopathic tinctures is the fresh plant, but parts of plants, barks, roots, seeds, gums, balsams, etc., are also used. Minerals and chemicals soluble in alcohol also give tinctures. When made from plants, it is essential to obtain the *fresh* flowering plant, whenever possible, the dried article always being inferior, often inert. For this reason, homœopathic tinctures must be imported from the country, where the plants, grow and *in no case will it answer to substitute a tincture made from the dried plant, or worse still, from a fluid extract.* It is very important that tinctures should be of uniform strength, and as the watery proportion varies greatly according to season and other conditions, the dried, crude drug is taken as the starting point from whence to calculate the strength of the tincture. This is readily ascertained by taking a suitable quantity of the fresh plant and weighing it, then drying it by gentle heat until there is no further loss of weight. The difference of weight will indicate the amount of water contained in the plant for which allowance is to be made in the use of the menstrua. But remember, that while the dry, crude material after evaporation is *taken as a unit of strength, the fresh green plant is to be used in the preparation of the tincture.*

The tincture represents one part of this dry, crude material in each ten parts of the completed solution, *i. e.*, 1x would represent its drug power. This is the method prescribed by the British and American Institute pharmacopœias, and leads to accurate and scientific results. At present, however, many tinctures are not made so and the mother tincture represents varying degrees of drug power, which ought to be known in each instance, in order to make an exact 1x attenuation.

Dilutions or Liquid Attenuations. Hahnemann introduced and adopted as the standard, a progressive scale of diluting drugs in the proportion of 1 to 99 known as the

Centesimal Scale. Under this rule each attenuation contains just $\frac{1}{100}$ part as much of the drug substance as the preceding attenuation. The potencies so prepared are marked 1, 2, 3, 4, etc., according to the potency represented. The first, 1, containing $\frac{1}{100}$ part of the crude drug, the second, marked 2, the $\frac{1}{100}$ part of the *first*, or $\frac{1}{10000}$ of the orginal drug; the third, marked 3, the $\frac{1}{100}$ of the second, or the $\frac{1}{1000000}$ of the original, etc. Later, in order to secure intermediate grades of strength and better communication of the particles, Hering introduced the

Decimal Scale, the proportion of 1 to 9 by which each successive dilution contains just $\frac{1}{10}$ as much of the drug substance as the preceding one.

Decimal preparations are designated such by an x; thus the first decimal is marked 1x, and contains $\frac{1}{10}$ part of the original drug substance; the second decimal is marked 2x, and contains the $\frac{1}{10}$ part of the first decimal, or $\frac{1}{100}$ of the original drug-substance. Thus it will be seen that the first *centesimal* is equal to the 2x; the 2nd centesimal, marked 2, is equal to the 4th decimal; the 3d centesimal to the 6x, etc., etc.

Triturations. A trituration is a preparation of a drug introduced by Hahnemann, by which the finely-powdered, medicinal substance is ground for a certain time in a mortar and pestle with a certain proportion of sugar of milk.

In the process of trituration, there is a progressive division and diminution of the medicinal substance, by which mechanical subdivision the visible particles of the substance become gradually smaller and fewer as the numbers of the triturations ascend—their surfaces are thereby immensely enlarged.

It can readily be seen that the surface occupied by a grain of any drug is greatly increased, if it can be divided into its constituent molecules. This can be done by triturating it with a larger quantity of some other substance—sugar of milk preferably—by which the distance between the molecules may be increased, and thus the surface extent enlarged. In this molecular form, the specific *quality* can be impressed upon the organism most effectually—for only in this form do the individual parts enjoy their freedom of motion, and can enter into the specific relations to the organism their affinity urges them on to. In the proportion as this molecular activity is attained, can these atoms enter the tissues of the body and there modify the functions.

To make Triturations. Hahnemann's method is still adhered to in all essential points, except that with the great increase of quantity required, most of the process of triturating is now done by means of machinery. At least one hour should be consumed to make each trituration and some drugs, especially in the first trituration, require a much longer time. The principle is taught clearly by Hahnemann. His original method was as follows:

Take 100 grains of fine sugar of milk and divide it into three equal parts; then add one grain of the drug to one of these three parts of sugar of milk in a mortar, mix well with a spatula, and then grind for six minutes with a moderate degree of force. The triturate is then to be scraped together for four minutes. Another third of sugar of milk is then added and treated exactly like the first third, and finally the last third is added and proceeded with in the same manner. This results in the first centesimal trituration (containing $\frac{1}{100}$ of the original drug). The second centesimal is made by taking one grain of the first and by proceeding with it in the manner described above. The third centesimal is made in the same manner from the second.

By adopting the decimal scale, a better preparation is ensured, since every centesimal trituration gets double the time of grinding, and this scale is therefore universally adopted.

All mineral preparations, most chemical salts, animal substances, and certain vegetable drugs and alkaloids, are thus prepared for purposes of homœopathy by first triturating them up to the sixth decimal or third centesimal potency. Each separate potency is triturated at least one hour, so the sixth has had no less than six hours constant triturating; but, as most triturations are now made by machinery, the time given to each is usually greatly extended. One hour, however, was Hahnemann's rule. Although many medicines have been carried up to the twelfth, and even the thirtieth potency, by *trituration*, there is no need or advantage in doing so beyond the sixth decimal, since Hahnemann proved conclusively, and clinical experience fully verified the fact, that beyond that potency all medicines yield up their medicinal virtues to water and alcohol, and can thus be prepared in a liquid state.

To Convert Triturations into Liquid Potencies. Hahnemann discovered the fact that any insoluble substance when triturated to the third centesimal or sixth decimal trituration, becomes so finely subdivided that its particles are held in suspension in the diluting menstruum, alcohol or water in other words are *practically* dissolved. In this way, all homœopathic medicines made from minerals and other insoluble substances are nevertheless converted into liquid preparations retaining all the medicinal virtues of the drug. The process is thus described by Hahnemann and adopted by the homœopathic profession:

"Sugar of Milk cannot be dissolved in pure Alcohol; this is the reason why the first dilution should be composed of one-half water and one-half alcohol. To one grain of the ($\frac{1}{1000000}$) third centesimal trituration, you add fifty drops of distilled water and turn the vial several times around its axis. By this means the Sugar of Milk becomes dissolved. Then you add fifty drops of Alcohol, and shake the vial. Only two-thirds of the vial ought to be filled with the solution." The vial is then marked with the name of the remedy and a figure 4, indicating the fourth centesimal potency. This preparation, containing one-half water cannot be used for saturating pellets as it would dissolve them. From this fourth the subsequent attenuations are made in the usual manner with pure alcohol. *

---

* One of the real dangers to Homœopathy consists in the lack of attention to the exact preparation of homœopathic medicines, and in substituting old school pharmaceutical methods for the precise and accurate instructions of Hahnemann. Dr. J. Hayward calls attention to this subject in a presidential address delivered in Liverpool last year. He says: "It is much to be feared, in view of the great competition and endeavor to undersell each other amongst the present-day homœopathic pharmacists, and with the low-priced tinctures, that many of the preparations are anything but those of genuine and pure drugs. This may be part of the cause of much of the disappointment we sometimes experience in practice. This risk is increased by the fact that many of our

Pellets, Disks, Cones, etc., are forms of vehicles for prescriptions. They are made of sugar and are simply saturated with the liquid attenuation. They are a convenient form of administering remedies.

Tablets are a compressed form of the trituration itself, of recent introduction. They come in one and two grain sizes, and are, therefore, very convenient when a definite size of dose is desired.

For further study consult the forthcoming Pharmacopœia of the American Institute of Homœopathy.

Also, "Three Lectures on Homœopathic Pharmaceutics," by the veteran pharmacist, Dr. F. E. Boericke.

---

drugs are procured from ordinary wholesale drug-stores, where they are not prepared with the care necessary for homœopathic medicines. It is very desirable that our own pharmacists should themselves collect and procure the medicines and make the preparations. If they will not, then practitioners should procure and prepare, at least, some of them for themselves."—(From a general survey of our position in *The Journal of the British Homœopathic Society*, January, 1896.)

CHAPTER XIII.

HAHNEMANN'S PHILOSOPHY.

Hahnemann was a vitalist. His philosophical conceptions are a protest against materialism; against all merely chemico-physiological ideas, all pathological, bacterial, antitoxic theories, discoveries and facts *as a basis for Therapeutics.* He proves that a true science of therapeutics cannot be built on any such insecure foundations, and the whole history of medicine justifies the position. Again, his teachings in regard to disease and their cure by homœopathic remedies require a practical acceptance of the existence of a vital principle animating the body, and at the same time a similar vital principle or force embodied in every medicinal substance. It necessitates therefore, a substantial world of causes, the world of mind where thought and affection, desire and lusts in their innumerable manifestations exist and a material world of effects, where these ultimate themselves in corresponding forms, and thus become fixed and enduring. Hahnemann saw in the body but an organism made up of material particles in themselves dead, but vivified and embodied and adapted to the real, living man, the spirit within. The connection between the immaterial, spiritual and immortal being, and the body is supposed by him to be effected by means of the vital force which he designates *Dynamis.* We have then, in Hahnemannian physiology, (1) the spirit, the true man, (2) the material body, receiving its life and health through (3) the vivifying vital force, the dynamis. From this conception follows the pathological deduction that the disturbance of the harmonious play of life, manifesting itself in symptoms affecting the functions and sensations which we call disease, is a disturbance of this same vital force or dynamis. This *Dynamis* differs from the material body in being of a more subtle quality and Hahnemann defines it, in contradiction of the material grossness of the body as "spirit-like." The vital force is active throughout the body, is the immediate cause of every functional activity, of all bodily growth. It is the *formative* force of the organism, is in fact the inner form which controls the molecular, chemical and mechanical processes, and uses them for its own purposes. Immaterial, hence beyond the penetration of the keenest sense or most powerful microscope, or the X ray. The vital force is the intermediate agent between the spirit and the body, enabling the spirit to dwell for a time in its material bodily clothing. Hahnemann's dynamis or vital force is not, therefore, the very seat of life, but only the connecting medium between the rational spirit, the true living man and the outer material covering by which man takes cognizance of this material world and its plane of external life. It is not necessary to suppose this vital force to be an organized entity, but rather the first ultimation on the plane of matter by means of the finest degrees of that plane, of the moulding, organizing and maintaining activity of the spirit within. If you choose to call it molecular motion, well and good, it is molecular motion guided for a definite end in view.

In disease, the vital principle is first disturbed, and its disturbance precedes functional and organic changes. *Hence, disease is of dynamic origin*, and the true causes of disease are such as affect the vital force; dynamic agents, mental conditions, passions, moral deteriorations in the individual or in the race. So-called causes of disease can act only as secondary causes when the vital force has become weakened in its resistance and allows untoward influences to affect the organism.

The following paragraphs in the Organon clearly teach this: 9, 10, 11, 12, 15, 16, 29.

"During health, the immaterial vital principle which animates the material body, rules absolutely. By it all its parts are maintained in admirable, harmonious vital operation, as regards both sensations and functions; so that our indwelling, rational spirit can freely employ this living, healthy instrument for the higher purposes of our existence."

"The material organism, without the vital force, is incapable of sensation, function or self-preservation; it is dead and subject only to the physical laws of the external world; it decays, and is again resolved into its chemical constituents; it is the immaterial, vital principle only, animating the material organism in health and disease, that imparts to it all sensation and enables it to perform its functions."

"In disease, it is only this immaterial, automatic vital force, pervading the entire organism, that is primarily deranged by the dynamic influence upon it of a morbific agent inimical to life. Only the vital principle, thus deranged, can furnish the organism its abnormal sensations and set up the irregular processes we call disease; for, as a power invisible in itself and only known by its effects on the organism, its morbid derangement only makes itself known by the manifestations of disease in the sensations and functions of those parts of the organism exposed to the senses of the observer and physician—that is, by *morbid symptoms*, and in no other way can it make itself known.

"How the vital force causes the organism to display morbid phenomena—that is, *how* it produces disease,—it would be of no practical utility to know, and, therefore, it will for ever remain concealed from the physician."

In the preface to the second volume of the "Materia Medica Pura," Hahnemann says: "Life is in no respect governed by any physical law which govern only inorganic substances. The material substances comprising the human organism are not governed in their living composition, by the same laws to which inorganic substances are subjected, but follow laws peculiar to their vitality; they themselves are animated and vivified, just as the whole organism is animated and vivified. * * * * As the organism, in its normal condition, depends only on the state of the vitality, it follows that the changed condition which we call disease or sickness must likewise depend, not on the operation of physical or chemical principles, but on originally vital sensations and actions—that is to say, a dynamically changed state of man—a changed existence, through which, eventually, the constituent parts of the body becomes altered in their character, as is rendered necessary in each individual case through the changed condition of the living organism."

Need of the Dynamized Remedy to Affect Changes in the Disturbed Vital Force. Now the next step was almost inevitable. If disease is but a disturbed condition of the vital force, and this far removed from the grossness of matter, so fine as to be almost spirit-like, surely crude drugs cannot possibly affect it curatively, and hence the need for purposes affecting this disturbed dynamis of the *dynamized* drug of the potentized remedy, one from which all crude, grossly material parts have been eliminated. * Such a prepara-

* The following quotation from Paracelsus is interesting in this connection, and may possibly serve as a clue to explain the action of the attenuated homœopathic medicines.

"Matter is connected with spirit by an intermediate principle which it receives from the spirit. This intermediate link between

tion alone would approach in character and fineness that of the dynamis, hence the teaching in Organon, 16, 269, 275, 276, 288, where it is said that it is only by means of the spirit-like influence of a morbific agent that our vital power can be diseased; and in like manner, only by the spirit-like (dynamic) operation of medicine that health can be restored.

"The homœopathic system of medicine develops for its use, to a hitherto unheard-of degree, the spirit-like medicinal powers of the crude substances by means of a process peculiar to it and which has hitherto never been tried, whereby only they all become penetratingly efficacious and remedial, even those that in their crude state give no evidence of the slightest medicinal power on the human body." § 256 Organon.

Hahnemann discovered the fact that there existed a dynamic, vital principle in all drugs, a curative force, peculiar and individual and distinctive of each drug, that could be *practically* transferred to some medicinally inert substance and preserved indefinitely. This is not saying that it becomes separated from its material basis, but the particles of this material envelope, if present at all, must be capable of a subdivision infinitely beyond that accepted by modern science.

A drug as we preceive it, is the *ultimate embodiment* of a medicinal force, differing in kind and degree in every drug, and Hahnemann devised or accidently hit upon a method, probably the only practical method, of securing this inner, living, medicinal force for therapeutic purposes.

---

matter and spirit belongs to all three kingdoms of nature . . . and it forms, in connection with the vital force of the vegetable kingdom, the Primum Ens, which possesses the highest medicinal properties." (Paracelsus).

The same thought is expressed in the following extract of a lecture on the Evolution of Medicine by Prof. Thos. J. Gray, M. D., of Minneapolis.

"We say that Opium is obtained from the Papaver Somniferum, Pulsatilla from the Anemone, Belladonna from the Atropa Belladonna, and so following. Just what do we mean in these statements? What is Opium or Pulsatilla or Belladonna? These plants named will grow and come to perfection in the same square foot of earth, in the same season, under the same conditions of air, light, soil, heat and moisture, yet each retains its identity; there is no transfer of individuality, each remains itself. Each has transmuted the common environment into himself, without any confusion or mistake. Upon closer examination, not alone do we find a common environment, but the microscope reveals an essential identity in structure. The protoplasmic vegetable cell is, so far as we can see, the same in them all, nay more, though our subtlest methods of chemical analysis must be confessed as crude approaches to the inner sanctuary of nature's secrets, since in the very nature of the case we cannot know the essential changes produced upon the original substances by our solutions and calexes, and so must furnish from the imagination long links of connecting conditions, yet they all point to an essential unity of chemical composition as well. If we reason on the plane of our experiments and observations, we are obliged to assume that the slight differences in structure and composition that seem to be present, are sufficient to account for one of the most stupendous facts in the natural world, a clear case of laying too heavy a burden on the major premise of the syllogism. But still more, when we contemplate the hidden processes by which the various vegetable cells unerringly appropriate and assimilate the common air, water and soil, in certain fixed proportions, do we see the force of this fact. Is it not a mere figure of speech to call the *form* in space of green and other colors, which appears to the eye, or whose reality may be attested by the balance, that space-filling and time-perduring thing, *the plant*, rather is it not a body for the real plant, the real thing, the thing that has caused what we can see and feel? This real poppy, this real anemone, or deadly night-shade, evidently is neither red or black, neither short or long, neither heavy or light, neither penetrable or impenetrable—in short, it *has not nor can have attributed to it any of the forms or qualities of bodies whatsoever.* Hence, it cannot be measured or weighed, nor can the terms much or little be applied to it. The poppy is as truly in one seed as in a thousand. *It is a dynamic energy, a force and not matter at all,* unless we make the confusion of assuming matter and force to be one and the same thing. And so of every drug, each is an active dynamic self. We acknowledge this truth in the phrase,'the active principle of this or that substance.'

And so it comes about that what we really administer is a principle, a force; a thing of which absolutely no attributes of matter can be predicated."

The keynote to Homœopathy is the Hahnemannian teaching of the Dynamis or vital force. Homœopathy eliminates material causes of most diseases, material dosage of medicines and looks to the real cause of all disease in the disturbed vital force and selects a curative remedy corresponding to all the symptoms expressing the disturbance and administers it in a dynamized form, one in which the drug is free to all outward appearance of its proper material envelope. This view of disease does not countenance therefore, a removal of the *products* of a disease as a cure of the disease itself, any more than blowing and cleaning of the nose is a cure for coryza. Hence the mere excision of tumors is no permanent cure of the tumor disease. We must go back of the local *manifestation* and cure the condition which produced the tumor. Local astringent injections do not cure a leucorrhœa, although the discharge is made to disappear; cauterizing a chancre will not cure the syphilitic cause of that outward manifestation of a general infection; a Sulphur or Zinc ointment applied to a skin disease, or a corrosive sublimate wash does not *cure*, although the skin itself may be freed. These measures merely suppress the local and ultimate manifestation of the disease. Metastases (change in the seat of disease), are sure to appear sooner or later and invariably more serious than tbe primary disorder. To be sure, the physician pronounces these new diseases, and the patient submits to further suppression and palliation, but a *cure* is further off than ever. Bear in mind that it is a fallacy to believe that disease can be cured by the expulsion of material morbific matters—they cannot be so permanently cured, though of course, the immediate symptoms of discomfort of the patient may be thereby removed. The physician's duty therefore, is more than to be a medical scavenger, expelling supposed or real morbific matter. There is no question that the loathsome, vile or impure discharges in diseases are effete *products* of the disease itself, symptoms of the dynamic disturbance within and as such guides to the selection of the remedy not to be carelessly suppressed, for frequently they are a relief of the inner more dangerous evil. By suppressing these outer manifestations, curative efforts of nature, possibly, metastases towards other and more vital parts are likely to take place.

For further study consult Chapter X, "Dynamization;" also, Chapter X on "Hahnemann's Doctrine of Chronic Diseases."

"The Genius of the Homœopathic Healing Art;" preface to the second volume of the Materia Medica Pura by Hahnemann.

Teste's Materia Medica; introductory chapter.

APPENDIX.*

A CATECHISM ON SAMUEL HAHNEMANN'S ORGANON.

A plain laborer went once to church to hear a celebrated preacher, whose eloquence was known near and far. After the service a parishioner asked that man how he enjoyed the sermon, and the poor man replied that it must have been a great sermon, but he failed to understand it. Years ago I gave to one of my students the Organon in vernacular and in the original to read, and bye and bye he came back and in sorrow exclaimed: "Why could that great man not write in such a language that a plain fellow, like me, can know what he meant?" Commentators tried over and over to explain every sentence (none better than Kent), and still the very necessity of commentators prove the necessity of abbreviating this great work, to give to the student the kernel in as few words as possible. If this is a sacrilege to the name of the father of homœopathy, may the good Lord pardon my sin.

---

* Some years ago, when the author edited the *California Homœopath*, the late Professor Samuel Lilienthal contributed to the journal a series of articles embodying the gist of Hahnemann's "Organon" and of his "Chronic Diseases" in simple language and especially written for the student. They were greatly appreciated at the time and repeated requests for their republication have been made. In compliance thereto and especially, as Professor Lilienthal's presentation is wholly in harmony with the purpose of this compend, the author believes that he will render a service to his readers and students generally, by enriching his pages with them.

1. The physician's highest and *only* calling is to restore health to the sick, which is called healing.

2. Healing ought to be accomplished in the most speedy, most gentle, and most reliable manner.

3. To do this he must know the ailment of the patient, select the remedy, the dose and its repetition according to each individual case.

4. Sanitation and hygiene are studies in which every physician must be well versed.

5. Constitution of the patient, his mind and temperament, occupation, mode of living and habits, social and domestic relations, age and sexual functions, etc. Give us the *individuality of the patient.*

6. Deviations from the normal state show themselves by morbid signs or symptoms.

7. The totality of these symptoms, *this outwardly reflected image of the inner nature of the diseased state, i. e., of the suffering dynamic, or living force*, is the principal and only condition to be recognized in order that they may be removed and health restored.

8. Life, a dynamic principle, animates the material body, and this material body passes away as soon as it is bereft of this life-force. In health, harmonious vital processes go on in our mind and body, and in sickness this life-force becomes deranged by the dynamic influence of some morbific agency inimical to life, hence abnormal functional activity, manifesting itself by morbid sensations and functions, by morbid symptoms.

9. This morbidly changed life-force can only be restored to its normal state by a similarly acting dynamical power of the appropriate remedy, acting upon the omnipresent susceptibility of the nerves of the organism. The total removal of all symptoms is health restored, and therefore the totality of symptoms observed in each individual case can be the only indication to guide us in the selection of a remedy.

10. These aberrations from the state of health can only be removed by the curative power inherent in medicine to turn the sensorial condition of the body again into its normal state.

11. Experiments on animals, vivisection and autopsy can never reveal the inherent power of medicine; the healthy human body alone is the fit subject for such experiments, where they excite numerous definite morbid symptoms, and it follows that, if drugs act as curative remedies, they exercise this curative power only by virtue of altering bodily failings through the production of peculiar symptoms, which then they are able to remove from the sick; in other words, the remedy must be able to produce an artificial morbid condition similar to that of the natural disease.

12. Experience teaches that all drugs will unexceptionally cure diseases the symptoms of which are as similar as possible to those of the drugs, and leave none uncured.

13. Natural diseases are removed by proper medicines, because the normal state is more readily affected by the right dose of a drug than by natural morbific agencies.

14. Psychical and partly physical terrestial potencies show their greatest power where this life-power is below par, hence they do not affect everybody nor do they do so at all times; we may therefore assert that extraneous noxious agencies possess only a subordinate and conditional power, while drug-potencies possess an absolute, unconditional power.

15. Drug-disease is substituted for the natural disease, when the drug causes symptoms most similar to that which is to be cured, and it is hardly possible to perform a cure by means of drugs incapable of producing in the organism a diseased condition similar to that which is to be cured.

16. Palliation of prominent symptoms ought to be discarded, for it provides only in part for a single symptom; it may bring partial relief, but this is soon followed by a perceptible aggravation of the entire disease.

17. Primary and after or counter effect of drugs. During the primary effect of a drug the vital force receives the impression made upon it by the drug and allows the state of health to be altered by it. The vital force then rallies and either calls forth the exact opposite state of feeling or it neutralizes the impression made upon it by the drug, thereby establishing the normal state of health. The former a counter effect, the latter a curative effect.

18. Diseases peculiar to mankind are of two classes: (1). Rapid, morbid processes caused by abnormal states and derangements of the vital force, *acute diseases*. (2). *Chronic diseases*. Originating by infection with a chronic miasm, acting deleteriously upon the living organism and undermining health to such a degree that the vital force can only make imperfect and ineffectual resistance, which may result in the final destruction of the organism.

19. Acute diseases may be sporadic, endemic or epidemic.

20. Allopathy is to blame for many an incurable ailment; the organism becomes gradually and abnormally deranged, according to the individual character of the drug.

21. True chronic diseases arise mostly from Syphilis, Sycosis and Psora. The latter is often the fundamental cause and source of countless forms of diseases, figuring as peculiar and definite diseases in our text-books on pathology.

22. *Individualization in the investigation of a case of disease* demands unbiased judgment, sound senses, at-

tentive observation and fidelity in noting down the image of the disease.

23. The patient tells the history of his complaints, the attendants fill out the gap, narrating every thing which he might have forgotten. *The physician observes by means of sight, hearing and touch* what is changed and abnormal about the patient, and writes down everything in precisely the same expressions used by the patient, and his attendants. Symptoms ought to be noted separately, one beneath the other, so that additions could be inserted. Careful inquiry by the physician will bring out the particular points, the modalities of each symptom. No leading questions are to be made, so that the patient may give unbiased his own sensations. Memoranda are then to be added of what he himself observed on the patient and anamnesis fully noted down.

24. The previous use of drugs may tarnish the picture of the disease, and it may be advisable to give a placebo for a day or two, so that afterwards a true picture may be attained. This holds specially good in chronic affections. In acute cases which brood no delay, the physician may be obliged to accept the morbid state as modified by drugs and embrace it in one record.

25. In chronic cases all the circumstances of the patient must be investigated: occupation, habits of living, diet, domestic relations, etc., so that appropriate means be taken for their removal. All this takes time and patience, as many chronic patients consider many a symptom as a part of their unavoidable condition, and forget to mention it, considering such of no value.

26. In the exploration of the totality of symptoms of epidemic or sporadic diseases, the physician should pre-suppose the true image of any prevalent disease to be new and unknown, and give it a new and thorough investigation. Nothing must be taken for granted.

In all epidemics the physician may only be able to collect the full picture of the disease after the investigation of several cases. Only thus he arrives at the characteristic peculiarities of the epidemic, which affects all patients *alike,* because each case arises from the same source, and then we are enabled to discover the appropriate homœopathic remedy for that prevailing epidemic.

27. When all the prominent and characteristic symptoms of the case have been committed to writing, the most difficult part has been accomplished, and we must now seek out the corresponding drug which in its effects on healthy persons produces symptoms strikingly similar to those of the disease. Upon subsequent inquiry concerning the effects of the remedy and the changes of feelings it has produced in the patient, and after having made a new record of the case, the physician only omits from his diary the symptoms which were improved, and notes down what remains, or what has subsequently appeared in the form of new symptoms.

28. The entire range of disease-producing power of each drug must be known, that is, all morbid symptoms and changes of the state of health which each drug is capable of producing by itself in *healthy persons,* in order to discover what elements of disease each is able to produce and inclined to excite by itself in the condition of mind and body. Thus, the disease-producing power of drugs can be made available homœopathically in the case of all diseases.

29. Experiments made with moderate doses of drugs (except narcotics, which destroy sensibility and sensation), upon healthy persons, exhibit only primary effects, *i.e.,* those symptoms by means of which a drug affects or deranges the healthy state and produces in the organism a morbid condition of variable duration.

30. *Some symptoms are produced by drugs in many healthy persons who try them; others are produced in only a few; others again are extremely rare,* showing themselves only in peculiar constitutions, which, though otherwise healthy, are inclined to be more or less morbidly affected by certain things which appear to make no impression and to produce no change in many other persons.

31. Each drug manifests particular effects in the human body, and no other drug will produce effects of exactly the same kind. Medicines must therefore be differentiated from each other with scrupulous accuracy, and proved by pure and careful experiments with regard to their power and true effects upon the healthy body. In proving drugs it should be remembered that strong, so called heroic substances, even in small doses, have the property of affecting changes in the health, even of robust persons. Those of milder power should be given in considerable doses in these experiments; and those of least activity, in order to cause their effect to become perceptible, should be tried only upon healthy, but sensitive and susceptible persons. Let us be very careful in regard to the reliability of the drugs used in the provings; they must be pure, genuine, and of full strength.

32. Every medicinal substance should be employed entirely alone, in a perfectly pure state, without the admixture of any other substance, and the prover should not take any other medicinal substance on the same day, or for so many days as the observation of the effects of the drug requires.

33. During the proving, the diet should be moderate, but nutritious; avoid all green vegetables, roots, all kinds of salad and pot-herbs, as they retain medicinal properties, even if most carefully prepared; avoid mental and bodily exertions, particularly disturbances

resulting from the excitement of sexual excesses. Provers ought to possess the requisite degree of intelligence to enable them to define, or to prescribe their sensations in distinct expressions.

34. Crude medicinal substances, if taken by the prover for the purpose of ascertaining their peculiar effects, will not disclose the same wealth of latent powers as when they are taken in a *highly attenuated state*, potentiated by means of trituration and succussion. Thus the medicinal powers, even of substances hitherto considered as inert, are most effectually developed by administering to the prover daily from four to six of the finest pellets of the thirtieth potency; the pellets, having been previously moistened with a little water, should be taken on an empty stomach for several days.

35. Drugs must be proved by both sexes, in order to get their full effects.

36. All persons differ in their susceptibility to drug influence. Each prover should begin with a small dose of medicine, gradually to be increased day by day where such a course appears proper and desirable.

37. By giving a sufficiently strong dose in the beginning of a proving, we get the exact, consecutive order in which the symptoms appear, and the prover can note the time at which each one appeared. Thus, we find out the genius of the drug. A moderate dose frequently suffices, when the prover is sensitive and pays proper attention to the state of his feelings. The duration of the effect of a drug is determined only after comparison of a number of provings.

38. When increased doses are taken several days in succession, we discover the various morbid conditions which this drug produces in general, but we will not learn the consecutive order of their appearance, and besides, a second dose, by its curative effect, will

often remove some of the symptoms resulting from the previous dose; or a second dose may produce the opposite condition from that of the first, an alternating effect of the drug.

39. An increased dose for several successive days shows the symptoms better, but not the consecutive order, nor the duration of the drug effect. During the proving the prover should study out whether any symptom is changed by taking different position, when ameliorated or aggravated, and at what time of day or night each symptom usually appears.

40. Several provings are necessary by the same prover to get from him as many symptoms as possible, but to get at the totality of symptoms which a drug is liable to produce, the provings of many persons are necessary; the smaller the dose of the drug, the more distinctly the primary effects will appear, while excessive doses cause the result to be disturbed by the appearance of various after-effects, because the primary effects become confused by the violence and haste of the action of the dose.

41. Symptoms similar to the drug the prover has sometimes felt before the proving was commenced, but when they appear again during the proving, it shows that he is susceptible to the action of the drug.

42. Every prover must be directed to distinctly write down every sensation and change of feeling, the time of its appearance, its duration, and then the director of the proving compares the different manuscripts of records. Thus, we accumulate a collection of genuine, pure, and undeceptive effects of simple drugs. Such records contain and represent in similitude the elements of numerous natural diseases hereafter to be cured by these means. A materia medica of that kind should exclude every supposition, every mere assertion or fiction.

43. A drug fully tested with regard to its power of altering human health, and whose symptoms present the greatest degree of similitude with the totality of symptoms of a given natural disease, will be the most suitable and reliable homœopathic remedy for that disease, its specific curative agent.

44. A medicine possessing the power to produce an artificial disease most similar to the natural disease to be cured, exerts its dynamic influence upon the morbidly disturbed vital force, and in the right dose will affect those parts of the organism where the natural disease is located, and will excite in them an artificial disease.

45. A well-selected homœopathic drug will remove a natural acute disease of recent origin, even if severe and painful; an older affection will disappear in a few days, and recovery progress to full restoration of health. Old, complicated diseases demand longer time for their removal. Chronic drug diseases, complicating an uncured natural disease, yield only after great length of time, if they have not become quite incurable.

46. For a few insignificant symptoms of recent origin, no medicinal treatment is needed; a slight change of diet and habits of living suffices for their removal.

47. In searching for the homœopathic specific remedy, the *more prominent, uncommon and peculiar* (characteristic) symptoms of the case should bear the closest similitude to the symptoms of the drug. The more general symptoms deserve less notice, as generalities are common to every disease and almost to every drug.

48. Although a well-selected remedy quietly extinguishes an analogous disease without exciting additional sensations, it may produce a slight aggravation resembling the original disease so closely that the pa-

tient considers it as such. Aggravations caused by larger doses may last for several hours, but in reality these are only drug effects somewhat superior in intensity and very similar to the original disease. The smaller the dose of the drug, so much smaller and shorter is the apparent aggravation of the disease during the first hours. Even in chronic cases, after the days of aggravation have passed, the convalescence will progress almost uninterruptedly for days.

49. If in acute cases the remedy was poorly selected we must examine the case more thoroughly for the purpose of construing a new picture of the disease. Cases may occur where the first examination of the disease and the first selection of the remedy prove that the totality of symptoms of the disease is not sufficiently covered by the morbific elements (symptoms) of a single remedy; and where we are obliged to choose between two medicines which seem to be equally well suited to the case, we must prescribe one of these medicines, and it is not advisable to administer the remedy of our second choice without a renewed examination of the patient, because it may no longer correspond to the symptoms which remain after the case has undergone a change, and often a different remedy will be indicated. If the medicine of our second choice is still suited to the remnant of the morbid condition, it would now deserve much more confidence and should be employed in preference to others.

50. Diseases presenting only a few symptoms may be called partial (one-sided) diseases; their chief symptoms indicating either an internal affection, or headache, or diarrhœa, or only a local one. A mere careful examination often reveals more occult symptoms, and if this fails, we must make the best use of these few prominent symptoms as guides in the selection of the medicine. As for such a partial disease, the selected

remedy may also be only partially adapted, it may excite accessory symptoms and symptoms of the disease will be developed which the patient had not previously perceived at all or only imperfectly, thus facilitating the task of selecting a more accurate homœopathic remedy.

51. After the completion of the effect of each dose of medicine, the case should be re-examined, in order to ascertain what symptoms remain and the corresponding remedy selected, and so on till health is restored.

52. Local diseases are those affections which are of recent origin and caused by external injury. *Affections of external parts, requiring mechanical skill, belong to surgery alone*, but often the entire organism is affected to such an extent by injuries, as to require dynamic treatment in order that it may be placed in the proper condition for the performance of the curative operation.

53. Affections of external parts, not caused by external injuries, proceed from an internal morbid state and all curative measures must be taken with reference to the state of the whole system, in order to effect the obliteration and cure of the general disease by internal remedies.

54. In examining such a case, the record of the exact state of the local disease is added to the summary of all symptoms, and other peculiarities to be observed in the general condition of the patient, in order to get at the totality of symptoms and to select the corresponding remedy which removes the local as well as the general symptoms. Notwithstanding the well-regulated habits of the patient a remnant of the disease may still be left in the affected part, or in the system at large, which the vital force is unable to restore to its normal state; in that case the acute local disease frequently proves to be the product of psora,

which has lain dormant in the system, where it is now about to become developed into an actual chronic disease. Antipsoric treatment will be necessary to remove this remainder and to relieve the habitual symptoms peculiar to the patient previous to the acute attack. (See Chronic Diseases.)

55. It is not advisable to combine the local application of a medicine simultaneously with its internal use, for the disappearance of the local symptom renders it nearly impossible to determine whether the total disease has also been exterminated by the internal remedy. Relying on the internal remedy alone, the removal of the local disease proves the achievement of a radical cure, and of complete recovery from the general disease.

56. When the system is affected with some chronic disease which threatens to destroy vital organs or life itself and which does not yield to the spontaneous efforts of the vital force, the latter endeavors to substitute a local disease on some external part of the body, whither the internal disease is transferred by derivation, in order to lessen the internal morbid process. But still the internal disease may increase constantly and their nature will be compelled to enlarge and aggravate the local symptoms in order to make it a sufficient substitute for, and to subdue the internal disease.

57. Most chronic diseases originate from three chronic miasma; internal syphilis, internal sycosis, and particularly from internal psora. Each of these must have pervaded the whole organism and penetrated all its parts before the primary representative local symptom makes its appearance for the prevention of the internal disease. The suppression of the local symptom may be followed by innumerable chronic diseases; the true physician cures the great fundamental miasm

together with which its primary as well as its secondary symptoms disappear together.

58. Before beginning the treatment of a chronic disease we must find out whether the patient ever had been infected by syphilis or by sycotic gonorrhœa, although it is rare to meet with uncomplicated cases of these affections, as we usually find them often complicated with *psora, the most frequent and fundamental cause of chronic diseases.* It will be necessary to inquire into all former treatment and what mineral .waters have been employed and with what result, in order to understand the deviations which the treatment had produced in the original disease, to correct this artificial deterioration and to determine the course now to be pursued.

59. A full anamnesis of the case ought now to be recorded, also the state of mind and temperament of the patient, as it may be useful to direct or modify this mental condition by psychical means. Guided by the most conspicuous and characteristic symptoms the physician will be enabled to select the first anti-psoric, anti-syphilitic or anti-sycotic remedy for the beginning of the cure.

60. The state of the patient's mind and temperament is often of most decisive importance in the selection of the remedy, as each medicinal substance affects also the mind in a different manner. Mental diseases must only be treated like all other affections and they are curable only by remedies similar to the disease.

61. Most mental alienations are in reality bodily diseases, only these mental and emotional symptoms develop in some cases more or less rapidly, assume a state of most conspicuous onesidedness, and are finally transferred like a local disease, into the invisibly fine organs of the mind, where they seem to obscure the bodily symptoms; in short, the disorder of the coarser

bodily organs are transferred, as it were, to the almost spiritual organs of the mind, where the dissecting knife will search in vain for their cause.

62. In recording the totality of symptoms of such a case, we must obtain an accurate description of all physical symptoms which prevailed before the disease degenerated into a one-sided mental disorder. We compare, then, these early symptoms with their present indistinct remnants, which occasionally appear during lucid intervals, and add the symptoms of the mental state as observed by the physician and attendants of the patient.

63. Though a patient may be relieved of an acute mental disorder by non-antipsoric medicine, no time must be lost in perfecting the cure by continued antipsoric treatment, so that the disease may not break out anew, which will be prevented by strict adherence to well-regulated diet and habits. If neglected, psora will be usually developed during the second attack, and may assume a form, periodical or continuous, and much more difficult to cure.

64. Mental diseases, not the result of physical or bodily affections, of recent date, and which have not yet undermined the physical health too seriously, admit of the speedy cure by physical treatment, while careful regulations of habits will re-establish the health of the body, but as a measure of precaution a course of antipsoric treatment is advisable, in order to prevent a recurrence of the attack of mental aberration. Proper hygiene and psychical regimen of the mind must be strictly enforced by the physician and attendants. *The treatment of insane persons should be conducted with a view of the absolute avoidance of corporeal punishment or torture. Physician and attendants should always treat such patients as if they regarded them as rational beings.*

65. Intermittent diseases also claim our attention. Some return at certain period, and there are others, apparently non-febrile affections, resembling intermittents by their peculiar recurrences. There are also affections characterized by the appearance of certain morbid conditions, alternating at uncertain periods with morbid conditions of a different kind. Such alternating diseases are mostly chronic and a product of developed psora, in rare instances they are complicated with syphilitic miasma. The first needs purely antipsoric treatment, the latter an alternation of antipsoric with antisyphilitics.

66. Typical intermittents recur after a certain period of apparent health, and vanish after an equally definite period. Apparently non-febrile morbid conditions, recurring at certain periods, are not of sporadic or epidemic nature, they belong to a class of chronic, mostly genuine psoric diseases. Sometimes an intercurrent dose of highly potentized Peruvian bark extinguishes the intermittent type of the disease.

67. In sporadic or epidemic intermittents, not prevalent endemically in marshy districts, each attack is mostly composed of two distinct stages, chill and heat. or heat and then chill; still more frequently they consist of three stages, chill, heat and finally sweat. The remedy, usually a non-antipsoric, must have the power to produce in healthy persons the several successive stages similar to the natural disease, and should correspond, as closely as possible, with the most prominent and peculiar stage of the disease; but the symptoms which mark the condition of the patient during the apyrexia, should chiefly be taken for guides in selecting the most striking homœopathic remedy. The best time to administer the medicine is a short time after the termination of the paroxysm, then the medicine has time to develop its curative effect without vio-

lent action or disturbance, and the vital force is then in the most favorable condition to be gently modified by the medicine and restored to healthy action. If the apyrexia is very brief, or if it is disturbed by the after effects of the preceding paroxysm, the dose of the medicine should be administered when the sweating stage diminishes or when the subsequent stages of the paroxysm decline.

68. One dose may suffice to restore health, but when a new attack threatens, the same remedy should be repeated, provided the complex of symptoms remains the same; but the intermittent is apt to recur, when the noxious influences, which first originated the disease, continue to act upon the convalescent patient, as would be the case in marshy localities, and to eradicate the tendency to relapses, the patient ought to be removed to a mountainous region. When this suitable remedy fails to break up the paroxysms, unless continued exposure to marsh miasma is at fault, we may blame the latent psora for it, and antipsoric remedies are needed for a cure.

69. Epidemics of intermittents in non-malarial districts partake of the nature of chronic diseases; each epidemic possesses a peculiar uniform character, common to all individuals attacked by the epidemic, and this uniform character points out the homœopathic remedy for all cases in general. This remedy usually also relieves patients, who, previous to this epidemic, had enjoyed good health, and who were free from developed psora.

70. In such epidemic intermittents our antipsorics fail, but a few doses of sulphur or hepar sulphur, repeated at long intervals, will aid us in their cure. Malignant intermittents, attacking single persons not residing in marshy districts, need in the beginning a non-antipsoric remedy, which should be continued for

several days, for the purpose of reducing the disease as far as possible. Where this fails, psora is sure in the act of development, and antipsorics alone will give relief.

71. Intermittent fevers, indigenous to marshy countries, or places subject to inundations, will hardly ever affect young and healthy people, *if their habits are temperate*, and if they are not weakened by want, fatigue or excesses. Endemics are apt to attack new comers, but a few doses of high potencies of China will easily rid them of the fever, provided their mode of life is very simple, and if there is no latent psora in them, which, where such is the case, necessitates antipsoric treatment.

72. *Mode of Application of Curative Remedies.*—Perceptible or continued improvement in acute or chronic diseases invariably counter-indicates the repetition of any medicine whatever, for every new dose would disturb the process of recovery. A very minute dose of the similimum, if uninterrupted in its action, will gradually accomplish all the curative effects it is capable of producing, in a period varying from forty to one hundred days. Yet physician and patient desire to reduce this period. We must be careful to select the most appropriate remedy, and then only we might repeat this potency in fourteen, twelve, ten, eight or seven days. In chronic diseases assuming an acute form, and demanding greater haste, these spaces of time may be abbreviated still more, but in acute diseases the remedies may be repeated at much shorter intervals, for instance, twenty-four, twelve, eight or four hours; and in the most acute cases at intervals varying from one hour to five minutes.

73. The dose of the same remedy is to be repeated, until recovery ensues or until the remedy ceases to produce improvement; and with the change of symptoms a fresh examination may indicate another remedy.

74. Every medicine which produces new and troublesome symptoms not peculiar to the disease to be cured, is not homœopathic to the case. An antidote must be given, selected with great care in regard to the similitude of the case, or if the accessory symptoms are not too violent, the next remedy should be given at once, in order to replace the inappropriate one. If in urgent cases we see after a few hours that the selection of the remedy was faulty and the patient fails to improve or new symptoms are discovered, we must select with greater care another remedy which is more accurately adapted to the new state of the case.

75. There are some remedies, as Ignatia, Bryonia, Rhus. rad., in some respects Belladonna, which show alternating effects on the state of the health, composed of partly opposite primary effects. If after the exhibition of one of these remedies, no improvement follows, we must in a few hours, in acute cases, give a new potency of the same remedy.

If in a chronic psoric case the antipsoric fails to relieve, there must be some irregularity of regimen or some other vigorous influence acting upon the patient, which must be removed before a permanent cure can be accomplished.

Incipient improvement, however slight, is indicated by increased sensation of comfort, greater tranquility and ease of the mind and return of naturalness in the feelings of the patient. To find out improvement or aggravation, the physician must examine the patient closely upon every symptom contained in the record of the case. If these show that neither new nor unusual symptoms have appeared, and that none of the old ones have increased, and especially if the state of mind and disposition is found to be improved, the medicine must also have produced an essential and general improvement in the disease, or at all events, it may soon be expected. Where delay occurs beyond expectation, there must be some fault in the regimen of the patient or the protracted homœopathic aggravation produced by the medicine must be attributed to the insufficient reduction of the dose.

76. New and important symptoms, mentioned by the patient, indicate that the medicine was not well selected; though the patient may think he is improving, his condition may even be worse, which will soon make itself apparent.

77. No physician should have favorites among drugs, nor should he disregard medicines on account of their failure. Too often the fault is the physician's or the supposition a wrong one; his only duty is to select the similimum to every case.

78. On account of the minuteness of the homœopathic dose, great care must be taken in the diet and regimen of the patient, and especially in chronic cases we have to search carefully for such impediments to a cure, because these diseases are often aggravated by obscure, noxious influences of that kind as well as by errors in regimen, which, being frequently overlooked, exercise a noxious influence. Daily walks, light manual labor, proper nutritious food and drink, unadulturated with medicinal substances are to be recommended. In acute cases we have only to advise the family to obey the voice of nature by gratifying the patient's ardent desires, without offering or urging him to accept hurtful things. In acute cases the temperature of the bedroom and the quantity of the covering should be regulated entirely according to the wishes of the patient, while every kind of mental exertion and emotional disturbance is to be avoided.

79. *Genuine and unadulterated medicines, retaining their full virtues* are the first requisites of a physician, and in the treatment of disease only *one single* medici-

nal substance should be used at one time; which will give relief in diseases whereof the totality of symptoms is accurately known. Too strong a dose, of even a well selected drug, will produce an unnecessary surplus of effect upon the over excited vital force, and will be injurious, while the same similar drug-disease, if exerted within proper limits, would have gently effected a cure.

80. Experience proves that the dose of a homœopathically selected remedy cannot be reduced so far as to be inferior in strength to the natural disease, and to lose its power of extinguishing and curing at least a portion of the same, provided that this dose, immediately after having been taken, is capable of causing a slight intensification of symptoms of the similar natural disease, though this homœopathic aggravation is very often almost imperecptible.

81. The homœopathic similimum will operate chiefly upon the diseased parts of the body, which have become extremely susceptible of a stimulus so similar to their own disease. The smaller dose will change the vital action of those parts into an artificial drug disease, and the organism be freed from the morbid process.

82. In homœopathic practice the diminution of the dose, and its effect is conveniently accomplished by lessening the volume of the dose. In using a solution of this kind a much greater surface supplied with sensitive nerves, susceptible of medicinal influence, is brought in contact with the medicine, and we must take care that the medicine is equally and intimately imparted to every particle of solvent fluid. The effect of medicines in liquid forms penetrates and spreads through all parts of the organism, with such inconceivable rapidity, from the point of contact with the sensitive nerves supplying the tissues, that this effect may, with propriety, be defined spirit-like or dynamic.

83. Remedies in their dynamic dose, may be given by the mouth and tongue, by olfaction, or hypodermically. The most sensitive parts of the surface are, at the same time, the most susceptible.

A CATECHISM ON THE FIRST VOLUME OF HAHNEMANN'S CHRONIC DISEASES.

1. All chronic diseases are so inveterate immediately after they have become developed in the system, that, unless they are thoroughly cured by art, they continue to increase in intensity until the moment of death. They never disappear of themselves, nor can they be diminished, much less conquered or extinguished, by the most vigorous constitution or the most regular mode of life and strictest diet.

2. Psora is the oldest, most universal and most pernicious chronic miasmatic disease. Existing for many thousands of years, its morbid symptoms have increased to such an extent that its secondary symptoms have become innumerable.

3. The ancient nations designated psora as leprosy, by which the external parts of the body became variously disfigured, and during the middle ages the Crusaders spread it over Europe. Cleanliness, increased refinement and more select nourishment succeeded in diminishing the disgusting appearance of psora so as to reduce the disease, towards the end of the fifteenth century, to the ordinary eruption of an itch. But about this time, 1493, the second contagious chronic disease, syphilis, began to raise its fearful head.

4. During the first centuries of leprosy the patients, though they suffered much in consequence of lanci-

nating pains in the tumors and scabs, and the vehement itching all around, enjoyed nevertheless a fair share of general health, for the obstinately lasting eruption upon the skin served as a substitute for the internal psora, and furthermore the leprous patients were kept apart from human society and thus the contagion remained limited and rare.

5. But the milder form of psora, in the shape of an itch, infected a far greater number of people, and the itch vesicles being constantly ruptured by scratching and their contents spread over the skin, and those things which had been touched by such patients, psora became the most contagious and most universal of the chronic poisons. Though this eruption by its easier concealment may attack many persons, still the essence of this reduced psora remains unchanged, and being more easily repelled from the skin, it appears so much more imperceptibly upon the inner surface, producing severe secondary ailments.

6. At the time before leprosy was reduced, there were much less nervous affections, painful ailments, spasms, cancerous ulcers, adventitious formations, weaknesses, paralysis, consumptions and degenerations of either mind or body, than there are now, aided probably by universal use of coffee and tea for the last two centuries.

7. The most universal of external means has done an immense amount of mischief, for secondary ailments will sooner or later manifest themselves as results of the psoric reaction.

8. Many cases from ancient and recent writers can be cited to convince the observer that the itch with its varieties, tinea capitis, crusta lactea, herpes, etc., are the external vicarious symptoms of an internal disease affecting the whole organism, and that psora is the most pernicious of all chronic poisons. It is well

known that all infections first attack the whole organism internally before the vicarious affection manifests itself.

9. In acute diseases, the local symptoms, together with the disease, leave the system as soon as they have run through their regular course. In chronic diseases the local affection may either be removed or disappear by itself, when at the same time the internal disease may increase, unless it is cured by art.

10. In considering the formation of the three chronic maladies, psora, sycosis, syphilis, as well as that of the acute infectious diseases, three cardinal points must be noticed: 1, the period when the infection took place; 2, the period when the whole organism began to be tainted with the infectious poison, until it became a complete internal disease; 3, the manifestation of the external symptoms, by which nature indicates the complete development of the infectious disease in the internal organism.

11. The infection in acute as well as in chronic diseases, takes place in a moment, provided this moment is favorable to the contagious influence; the whole nervous system becomes infected in a moment. The human small-pox, measles, etc., will run through their course, and the fever which is peculiar to each of these different forms of infection, together with the cutaneous eruption, will break out a few days after the internal disease has completed its development.

12. The mode of contagion in chronic contagious diseases is the same, but after the internal disease is completed, there is this difference, that the chronic poison continues in the organism, and even develops itself from year to year, unless it is extinguished and thoroughly cured by art.

13. Syphilitic contagion happens at those places which come in contact with the syphilitic virus and

receive it into themselves by friction; the internal organism is roused in a moment by this infection, and not until the internal disease is completely developed, does nature try to form at the spot where the contagion took place, a local symptom as a substitute for the internal disease. By extinguishing the internal disease with an internal remedy, the chancre becomes also cured without any external application.

14. Psora is the most contagious of all chronic diseases, as it taints the system, especially that of children, by simply touching the skin. Not till the whole organism has been adapted to the nature of the chronic contagious disease, do the morbidly affected vital powers try to alleviate the internal disease by local symptoms and the eruption is merely the ultimate boundary of the psoric development, a substitute for the internal disease, which, together with its secondary ailments, remains in a latent condition. External applications may check the local symptoms, but too often the internal psora is thus aggravated.

15. There are many symptoms that reveal the existence of psora, but they cannot all be found upon one person; one has more, the other less, in one they come out progressively, in another they remain suppressed; this depends greatly upon the constitution and the external circumstances of the patient. These affections do not prevent him from leading a tolerably comfortable existence, provided he is young and robust, is not obliged to fatigue himself, has all his wants provided for, is not exposed to chagrin or grief and has a cheerful, calm, patient and contented temper. In this case psora may continue slumbering for years without becoming developed into a permanent chronic disease.

16. However, a trival cause, an ordinary vexation, a cold, an irregularity in the diet, etc., may, in a more advanced age, cause a violent though short attack of

disease, out of proportion with the moderately exciting cause, especially during the fall, winter and early spring.

17. But whenever the vital power has been reduced by some mental ailments or by a bodily affection, the latent psora becomes aroused and develops a host of inveterate symptoms; some one of the psoric chronic diseases break forth, unless more favorable circumstances set in, diminishing the intensity of the disease and making its ulterior development more moderate. (Here follow the symptoms of the aroused psora, differing according to the individuality of the patient and the extent of the psoric intoxication.)

18. Sycotic excrescences are often accompanied with a sort of gonorrhœa from the urethra, are sometimes dry and in the form of warts, but more frequently soft, spongy, emitting a fetid fluid, of a sweetish taste, bleeding readily and having the form of a coxcomb or a cauliflower. In man they appear upon the glans and around or beneath the prepuce; in woman they surround the pudenda. Surgery and mercury are still much abused in sycosis; the extirpation of the excrescences only lead to their appearance at some other place and the internal use of mercurials rouses a latent psora and we deal then with a combination of psora and sycosis. Our duty then is to annihilate the psoric miasm by the indicated antipsorics, and then we use the remedies indicated for sycosis (Thuja, Nitric acid), and for syphilitic complications Mercury remains the remedy.

19. The syphilitic contagion is much more general than the poison of sycosis. The treatment of syphilis is only difficult when complicated with the psoric poison. The former is rarely complicated with sycosis, but whenever it exists we meet psora as an additional complication.

20. Chancre and bubo are the original representatives of syphilis, and if not interfered with, they might remain during life and no secondary symptoms will appear. By considering the chancre a mere local ulcer and by removing it by external means, the disease is forced to manifest itself throughout the organism with all the secondary symptoms of a fully developed syphilis; hence it is that the internal disease is most permanently cured while the chancre or the bubo are yet existing as its vicarious types, especially in young persons of a cheerful temper, where often one single minute dose of Mercury suffices, and Hahnemann prefers that preparation which goes by his name. If more than one dose should be required, the lower potencies may then be employed.

21. The second stage sets in when the chancre has been speedily removed by external means, but even then, provided there is no latent psora, the secondary symptoms may be prevented by the soluble Mercury, and the original spot of the chancre can no more be traced, while without that internal treatment a reddish morbid-looking, red or bluish scar remains. Bubo, when not complicated with psora, only needs the same treatment.

22. In the third stage we find syphilis complicated with psora and the patient suffered already from psora when the syphilitic infection took place or false internal and external treatment caused a combination of the psoric with the syphilitic element and it take then more than one remedy to remove the evil consequences. It may be here observed that it is the nature of the psoric poison to break forth in consequence of great concussions of the system and violent inroads upon the general health.

23. In order to reach this marked syphilis (pseudo syphilis), we must remove from the patient all hurtful

external influences and put him on an easily and vigorously nourishing diet and regulate his general mode of life. The most appropriate antipsoric must then be selected which may be followed by a second antipsoric according to the new symptoms, and when the latter has accomplished its action, the single dose of Mercury must be allowed to act as long as it is capable of exercising a curative influence.

24. In old difficult cases, ailments remain which are neither purely psoric or syphilitic. Here several courses of antipsorics are needed, until the last trace of all provocation has ceased. After this we give a lower potency of Mercury and allow it to act until the skin has recovered its healthy color at the spot where the venereal chancre stood.

25. A complication of the three chancre poisons must be treated on the same principles. Antipsoric first and then that poison whose symptoms are most prominent. Afterwards the remaining portion of the psoric symptoms must be removed and then the last traces of syphilis and sycosis by other adequate remedies. A return of a healthy color of the skin on places which had been affected, is the surest sign of a perfect restoration.

26. As long as the psora eruption is yet existing upon the skin, psora exhibits itself in its simple and most natural integrity, and may be cured in the easiest, quickest and safest manner; but when the internal disease is deprived of its vicarious symptoms, the psoric poison is forced to spread over the most delicate parts of the internal organism and to develop its secondary symptoms.

27. The psoric poison having pervaded millions of organisms for thousands of years, has gradually developed out of itself an endless number of symptoms, varied according to differences of constitution, climate, residence, education, habits, occupation, mode of life,

diet, and various other bodily and mental influences; herein different antipsoric remedies will be required for the eradication of the psoric poison.

28. Only the recent itch, with the eruption still existing upon the skin, can be completely cured by one dose of sulphur; but such a speedy cure is not always possible, as the age of the patient has great influence upon the result of the treatment. In eruptions which have existed for some time on the skin, it ceases to be a vicarious symptom for the internal disease, and secondary psoric affections will manifest themselves; in such case sulphur does not suffice, and it requires several antipsorics for a cure.

29. With rèlation to diet and mode of life, whatever is injurious to the action of the remedies must be avoided, and with lingering diseases we must consider the age, occupation and social conditions of the patient. Strict diet alone will hardly ever cure a disease, and it is unreasonable to insist upon a mode of life which is impossible for a patient to follow; only that which is generally injurious to health, ought to be carefully avoided.

30. Rich patients must walk more than they usually do; moderate dancing, rural entertainments, music and amusing lectures, theaters once in a while are allowable, but they must never play cards; riding horseback or in a carriage ought to be restricted. All amorous intercouse and sensual excitement, reading lewd novels, superstitious and exciting books, are to be carefully avoided.

31. The literary man ought to take much exercise in the open air; in bad weather do some light mechanical work in the house. During treatment he ought to limit his literary work, and in mental diseases reading must be positively forbidden.

32. Chronic patients must avoid domestic medicines and abstain from perfumes. Those who are ac-

customed to wear wool may continue to do so, but as the case progresses and the weather becomes warmer, cotton or linen ought to be substituted. Daily ablutions are often more advisable than baths.

33. In regard to eating, one should consent to restrictions in order to be freed from a troublesome chronic disease, and only in abdominal affections restrictions are more necessary. In regard to beverages, coffee has pernicious effects upon mind and body. Young people do not need it, and older persons ought to wean themselves generally from its use, and be satisfied with roast rye or wheat, whose smell and taste is very much like coffee. Tea ought tô be entirely avoided during treatment of chronic diseases. Old people cannot be suddenly deprived of their wine, but by mixing it with water and sugar, they can gradually reduce its strength; in fact, the patient cannot be too abstemious in relation to alcoholic beverages; it is a law of nature that the apparent increase of strength and animal heat consequent upon the use of ardent spirits will be followed by a state of depression and diminution of heat.

34. Beer is so much adulterated, that it becomes injurious to health; vinegar and lemon juice are especially hurtful to those who are affected with nervous and abdominal complaints; sweet fruits may be used moderately; beef, wheat or rye bread, cow's milk and fresh butter are the most natural food, hence also for chronic patients. Next to beef comes mutton, game, old chickens, young pigeons. Goose, duck, or pork are less admissible. Salt and smoked meats ought to be used in great moderation. Fish ought to be boiled and eaten without any spiced sauces; herrings and sardines in moderate quantities. Moderation in both eating and drinking is a sacred duty for all chronic patients.

35. Restriction in the use of tobacco is especially necessary when the intellectual functions are affected, when the patient does not sleep well, is dyspeptic and constipated.

36. Excessive fatigue, working in marshy regions, injuries and wounds, excessive heat or cold, starvation, poverty, unwholesome food are less capable of rousing latent psora or aggravating a manifest psoric disease than an unhappy marriage or a gnawing conscience. Grief and sorrow are the chief causes which either develop latent psora or aggravate an already existing secondary psoric affection.

37. Mineral springs and all medicinal influences ought to be avoided and when the patient used them, he ought to abstain for some time from all medicines and follow a strict diet in the country.

38. All excesses injure mind and body; by vicious practices the most robust bodies often fail and the latent psora entering in combination with a badly managed syphilitic poison gives origin to most distressing diseases. We must then remove first the psoric poison and thus prevent all secondary chronic affections.

39. The physician must never interrupt the action of an antipsoric remedy nor exhibit an intermediate remedy on account of every trifling ailment; a carefully selected remedy should act till it has completed its effect.

40. Suppose the remedy calls out symptoms which have existed before, this apparent aggravation and the development of new symptoms show that the remedy has attacked the disease in its inmost nature, and it must be left undisturbed.

41. Should the remedy cause new symptoms, which may be supposed to be inherent to the medicine, the remedy should be permitted to act for a while and

generally these symptoms will disappear; but if they are troublesome, they show that the remedy was not properly chosen, and an antidote, if known, must be given or another suitable antipsoric selected.

42. A homœopathic aggravation is a proof that a cure may be anticipated with certainty; but if the original symptoms continue with the same intensity, it shows that too large a dose made the cure impossible, neutralizing its genuine homœopathic effects and causing a medicinal disease by the side of the natural disturbances. We then select an antipsoric which corresponds to the symptoms of the natural and of the artificial disease. Should the same antipsoric be still indicated, we must give it in a much higher potency and in a more minute dose. The doses can scarcely be too much reduced, provided the effects of the remedy are not disturbed by improper food.

43. The physician ought to avoid three mistakes, that the dose can be too small, the improper use of the remedy, and in not letting the remedy act a sufficient length of time. The surest and safest way of hastening a cure is to let the medicine act as long as the improvement of the patient continues.

44. Psora is a troublesome thing to deal with, exacerbations show only that the disease is writhing under the action of the remedy, but they will progressively diminish in frequency and intensity if not interfered with by a new remedy, for the benign action of the former remedy, which was manifesting itself, is thus probably lost.

45. A second dose of the selected remedy is only indicated when the improvement which the first dose had produced, by causing the morbid symptoms gradually to become less frequent and less intense, ceases to continue after the lapse of fourteen, ten or seven days, when it is evident that the medicine has ceased to act;

the condition of the mind is the same as before, and no new or troublesome symptoms have made their appearance. It may be expedient to give this second minute dose in a somewhat lower potency.

46. Sulphur, hepar, and sepia excepted, the other antipsorics, seldom admit of a favorable repetition of the same drug. One antipsoric having fulfilled its object, the modified series of symptoms generally requires another remedy. In cases treated by the old school it may be necessary to interpolate, once in a while, a dose of sulphur or hepar, according to indications.

47. Alternating remedies in rapid succession is a sure sign that the right remedy was not selected, or that the symptoms were only carelessly studied. By such mismanagement remedial agents seem to lose all their power, and mesmeric action may succeed in calming the system. Let the palms of both your hands rest for about a minute upon the vertex, then move them slowly down the body, across the neck, shoulders, arms, hands, knees, legs, feet and toes; this pass may be repeated.

48. The irritability of the patient may also be calmed by directing him to smell a globule moistened with the highest potency of the homœopathic medicine. By smelling of the medicine, its influence may be communicated to the patient in any degree. By increasing the number of inspirations the power of the medicine steadily increases.

49. Globules, kept in corked vials, protected from heat and sunshine, preserve their medicinal powers for years.

50. Placebos are in order where the patient wishes to take medicine every day.

51. The cure of a chronic disease may be often retarded by bodily or mental accidents, or intercurrent diseases, due to malaria or meteoric influences, may set

in, interrupting the antipsoric treatment sometimes for several weeks, and olfaction of the non-antipsoric remedy may suffice for the removal of the intermediate disease.

52. After the intercurrent disease is removed, the symptoms of the original chronic disease may be modified or morbid symptoms may manifest themselves in other parts of the body. The patient must be thoroughly re-examined, so that the appropriate remedy may be chosen.

53. Great epidemic diseases, improperly treated and permitted to complete their course, arouse the latent psoric poison often to a high degree of intensity, manifesting itself in innumerable forms, and antipsoric treatment is the only safeguard.

54. The obstinate character of endemic diseases is due to some psoric complication or the action of the psoric poison modified by the peculiar influence of the locality and the peculiar mode of life of its inhabitants. The marshy exhalations, especially of hot countries, appear, on account of their paralyzing influence over the vital forces, to be one of the most powerful excitants of the psoric poison, which can only be calmed by antipsoric treatment. Recently developed symptoms are the first to yield to the action of the antipsorics, the older symptoms, which have permanently existed, are the last to disappear, hence local symptoms only pass off after the general health has been completely restored, and we must not be contented till the last vestige of psora is removed.

55. A great chronic disease may be cured in the space of one or two years, provided it was not mismanaged to the extent of having become incurable. In young robust persons half this space of time is sufficient. If we consider that the psoric poison has gradually ramified into the inmost recesses of the organism,

patient and physician understand why much time must be necessary to master this parasitical enemy that has assailed the most delicate roots of the tree of life.

56. Where antipsoric treatment is properly conducted, the strength of the patient increases from the start and this increase in strength continues during the whole treatment until the organism unfolds anew its regenerate life.

57. The best time for taking an antipsoric is the morning, before breakfast and the patient ought then to wait about an hour before eating or drinking anything.

58. Antipsorics should neither be taken immediately before nor during menstruation. If the menses appear too soon, too abundant, and last too long, she may smell on the fourth day of a globule of a high potency of nux vomica, and several days after the antipsoric may be taken. Nux restores the harmony of the nervous functions and calms that irritability which inhibits the action of the antipsoric.

59. Pregnancy offers a brilliant sphere of action to antipsoric remedies, but only the highest potencies ought to be employed. Nurslings ought to get their medicine through the milk of the mother or wet nurse.

60. The vital force, if left to itself, tries to palliate by producing secretions and evacuations, or diarrhœas, vomiting, sweats, ulcers, hemorrhages, etc., but they produce only an apparent alleviation of the primitive disease, and in fact increase it on account of the great loss of nutritious pabulum which the patient has suffered.

61. At the beginning of the antipsoric treatment constipation is often the great bugbear of the patient, and an injection of pure tepid water may be allowed, which may be several times repeated, until the anti-

psoric remedies succeed to regulate the proofs of intestinal evacuation. Sulphur and lycopodium act most favorably under those circumstances. Hot baths interfere with the effects of antipsoric treatment.

62. The smallest possible electrical sparks aid the antipsoric treatment by animating those parts of the body which had been long affected with paralysis or insensibility.

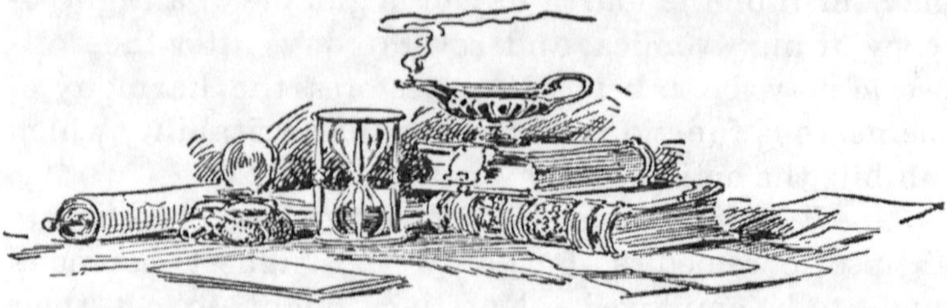

INDEX.